Cardiothoracic
Surgical Nursing
SECRETS

Cardiothoracic Surgical Nursing SECRETS

BARBARA A. TODD, MSN, CRNP
Director, Clinical Surgical Specialists and Practitioners
Department of Surgery
Hospital of the University of Pennsylvania
Philadelphia, Pennsylvania

SERIES EDITOR

LINDA SCHEETZ, EdD, APRN, BC, CEN
Assistant Professor
College of Nursing
Rutgers, The State University of New Jersey
Rutgers, New Jersey

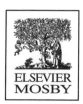

ELSEVIER
MOSBY

ELSEVIER
MOSBY

11830 Westline Industrial Drive
St. Louis, Missouri 63146

CARDIOTHORACIC SURGICAL NURSING SECRETS   ISBN 0-323-03267-2
Copyright © 2005, Mosby, Inc.

International Standard Book Number 0-323-03267-2

Executive Publisher: *Barbara Nelson Cullen*
Editor: *Sandra Clark Brown*
Developmental Editor: *Sophia Oh Gray*
Publishing Services Manager: *John Rogers*
Senior Project Manager: *Kathleen L. Teal*
Senior Design Project Manager: *Bill Drone*

Working together to grow
libraries in developing countries

www.elsevier.com | www.bookaid.org | www.sabre.org

ELSEVIER   BOOK AID International   Sabre Foundation

Printed in the United States of America

Last digit is the print number: 9 8 7 6 5 4 3 2 1

I would like to dedicate this book to all my family, friends, colleagues, and patients who have taught me many lessons.

Contributors

V. PAUL ADDONIZIO, M.D.
Chief, Division of Cardiac Surgery
Abington Memorial Hospital
Abington, Pennsylvania

Professor of Surgery
Temple University
Philadelphia, Pennsylvania

NANCY P. BLUMENTHAL, MSN, CS, CRNP
Instructor
University of Pennsylvania
School of Nursing
Philadelphia, Pennsylvania;

Senior Nurse Practitioner
Lung Transplant Program
University of Pennsylvania Medical Center
Philadelphia, Pennsylvania

DONNA CHOJNOWSKI, MSN, CRNP
Clinical Manager, Heart Failure Nurse Practitioner
Heart Failure, Heart Transplant Program
Hospital of the University of Pennsylvania
Philadelphia, Pennsylvania

SANDRA DAVIS, MSN, CRNP
Assistant Professor
Drexel University
Philadelphia, Pennsylvania;

Nurse Practitioner, Cardiothoracic Surgery
Abington Memorial Hospital
Abington, Pennsylvania
    3. Hypertension
    12. Preoperative Evaluation

KIMBERLY ANN DEVINE, RN, MSN, CRNP-CS, CCRN
Clinical Research Coordinator, Nurse Practitioner
Saint Mary Medical Center
Langhorne, Pennsylvania
    4. Dyslipidemia
    5. Coronary Artery Disease

KRISTAN MARIE DEVINE, RN, MSN, CRNP-CS, CCRN
Nurse Practitioner, Cardiac Surgery
Abington Memorial Hospital
Abington, Pennsylvania
    10. Pericardial Disease
    11. Congenital Heart Disease
    13. Hemodynamic Monitoring and Vasoactive Medications

THERESA HOLLANDER, PhD, RN, CS, CCTC
Mechanical Assist Device Coordinator/Research Coordinator
Temple University Hospital
Philadelphia, Pennsylvania
    17. Cardiac Transplantation
    18. Ventricular Assist Devices

JANICE JONES, RN, MSN, CPNP
Nurse Practitioner
Pennsylvania Cardiology Associates
Philadelphia, Pennsylvania
    15. Coronary Artery Bypass Grafting
    22. Thoracic Surgical Procedures
    24. Management of the Postoperative Thoracic Surgery Patient

ANNE MARIE KUZMA, RN, MSN, CTTC
Lead Lung Transplant/Pulmonary Nurse Coordinator
Temple University Hospital
Philadelphia, Pennsylvania
    21. Pulmonary Disorders

ANNETTE MITCHELL, MSN, RN, CCRN, CRNP
Cardiovascular Nurse Practitioner
Thomas Jefferson University Hospital
Philadelphia, Pennsylvania
   8. Cardiac Arrhythmias

VALENTINO PIACENTINO III, PhD
Post-Doctoral Fellow/Medical Student
Temple University School of Medicine
Philadelphia, Pennsylvania
   1. Cardiac Anatomy
   2. Cardiac Physiology

GERALD T. RANKIN, BA, BSN, RN, CCRN
Registered Nurse
Abington Memorial Hospital
Abington, Pennsylvania
   20. Emergent Bedside Sternotomy

SUSAN BAKER SAMPLE, MSN, CRNP
Nurse Practitioner
VAD Coordinator for Cardiac Surgery
Lancaster General Hospital
Lancaster, Pennsylvania
   19. Management of the Postsurgical Patient with Cardiac Disease

SCOTT A. SCHARTEL, DO
Professor of Anesthesiology, Residency Program Director
Temple University
Philadelphia, Pennsylvania
   14. Anesthesia for Cardiac Surgery

KATHLEEN SHAUGHNESSY, RN, MSN, CRNP
Nurse Practitioner, Cardiac Surgery
Abington Memorial Hospital
Abington, Pennsylvania
   7. Aortic Dissection
   20. Emergent Bedside Sternotomy

ROSE SHAFFER, RN, MSN, ACNP-CS, CCRN
Cardiology Nurse Practitioner
Thomas Jefferson University Hospital
Philadelphia, Pennsylvania
   8. Cardiac Arrhythmias

KAREN R. STEINKE, RN, MSN
Lung Transplant Coordinator
Temple University Hospital
Philadelphia, Pennsylvania
21. Pulmonary Disorders

BARBARA A. TODD, MSN, CRNP
Director, Clinical Surgical Specialists and Practitioners
Department of Surgery
Hospital of the University of Pennsylvania
Philadelphia, Pennsylvania
6. Valvular Heart Disease
16. Valvular Heart Surgery

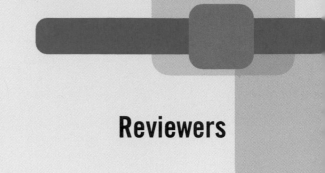

Reviewers

RONALYN CHAPLEAU, RN, BSN, MSN
Registered Nurse
Divisional Support Department
All Saints Healthcare, St. Mary's Medical Center
Racine, Wisconsin

DESIREE A. FLECK, MSN, CCRN, CPNP
Nurse Practitioner/Coordinator
Cardiac Center/Adult Congenital Heart Disease Center
The Children's Hospital of Philadelphia
Philadelphia, Pennsylvania

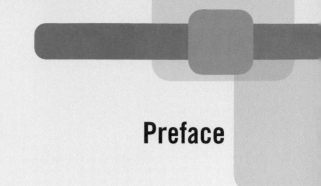

Preface

Throughout several years spent as an advance practice nurse in cardiothoracic surgery, I have learned many lessons from my colleagues as well as from patients. I continue to be intrigued about the dynamic nature of the discipline.

This book is intended to be a quick reference for the nurse involved in the care of cardiothoracic surgery patients. The chapters in the book are a review of current information related to a specific topic and selected concepts related to cardiothoracic care. This book is divided into cardiac and thoracic topics. It is not meant to be inclusive of all the problems that may confront the clinician. Top Secrets have been identified for each chapter, as well as for the entire text.

I would like to acknowledge the authors that contributed their knowledge and time to this book and who continue to participate in the care of cardiothoracic surgery patients.

I would like to thank my family, friends, and colleagues for their support of this project. Also, I would like to thank Linda Scheetz and the Elsevier staff for their guidance on this project, and helping me persevere to completion.

The success of this project will depend on the ability to be helpful to the readers.

BARBARA A. TODD

Contents

Top Secrets

1. Right coronary artery occlusion often presents with bradyarrythmias and heart block.
2. Cardiac murmurs are graded on a scale of one to six.
3. All diastolic murmurs are pathologic of disease.
4. Systolic murmurs may be innocent.
5. Blood pressure is influenced by systemic vascular resistance (SVR) and cardiac output.
6. A complete lipoprotein profile should be done at age 20 and every 5 years thereafter.
7. Esophageal spasm may mimic angina pectoris and be relieved with nitrates.
8. Intra-aortic balloon pumping (IABP) is contraindicated in patients with moderate to severe aortic insufficiency.
9. Administer vasodilators cautiously in patients with aortic stenosis.
10. Coronary artery bypass grafting is recommended in patients with significant left main stenosis and cardiogenic shock.
11. Patients being discharged after myocardial infarction should have prescriptions for aspirin, beta-blockers, ACE inhibitors, Plavix, and cholesterol-lowering agents, unless contraindicated.
12. Atypical symptoms of angina may include fatigue, congestive heart failure, and flu-like symptoms.
13. In a patient with suspected aortic dissection, blood pressure should be measured on all extremities.
14. Syncope, angina and dyspnea are the most common symptoms associated with aortic stenosis.
15. Rheumatic fever is the most common cause of mitral stenosis.
16. After surgery for mitral regurgitation patients will have a reduction in the left ventricular ejection fraction.
17. A widened pulse pressure is seen in patients with chronic aortic regurgitation.
18. Heart block is the most common arrhythmia after aortic valve surgery.
19. Increasing sternotomy pain may be the first clinical signs of mediastinitis.
20. Patients on cardiac telemetry should be monitored in lead V1.
21. Atrial fibrillation is commonly associated with mitral valve disease.
22. The surgical MAZE procedure is utilized to treat chronic atrial fibrillation.
23. Hypertension control is very important in the treatment of aortic dissections and aneurysms.
24. Cardiac transplantation survival has improved with newer immunosuppressive agents.
25. Atrial fibrillation after cardiac transplantation may be the first sign of allograft rejection.
26. Mechanical assist devices have improved the survival rate of patients awaiting cardiac transplantation.

27. Patients with fixed irreversible pulmonary hypertension are not candidates for cardiac transplantation.

28. A chylothorax is usually caused by trauma to the lymphatic system.

29. If a new airleak in a chest tube drainage system occurs, please rule out loose connections.

30. The best treatment for pulmonary embolus is prevention.

31. Coarctation of the aorta is one of the causes of secondary hypertension.

32. Hypercarbia is a prognostic indicator of the patient's pulmonary risk for undergoing thoracic surgery.

33. Hemoptysis may be the first sign of a pulmonary artery rupture.

34. Large "V" waves are indicative of mitral regurgitation.

35. Thiocynate toxicity may occur from prolonged nitroprusside use.

36. Endocarditis may occur early and late after valvular heart surgery.

37. The treatment for tricuspid valve endocarditis is usually antibiotics.

38. Dental evaluation should be done on all patients before valvular heart surgery.

39. Cardiac tamponade may occur after the removal of the epicardial pacer wires.

40. The role of the nurse is very important in the event of an emergency bedside sternotomy.

41. Patients with left to right shunts will usually present with pulmonary hypertension and congestive heart failure.

42. Patients with diabetes and coronary artery disease may have silent ischemia.

43. Early extubation after cardiac surgery leads to decreased pulmonary morbidity.

44. Pain control after thoracic surgery is important in order to decrease pulmonary complications.

45. Hypothermia may lead to increased bleeding in patients after cardiac surgery.

46. Atrial fibrillation in the postoperative period is best treated with betablockers.

47. Wean inotropes in postoperative cardiac surgery patients systematically.

48. Monitor serum glucose levels closely in patients on epinephrine drips.

49. Placement of the transesophageal probe during cardiac surgery may be associated with pharyngeal, esophageal, and gastric injury.

50. Coronary bypass grafting is being done increasingly without the use of the heart lung machine.

Cardiovascular

Chapter 1

Cardiac Anatomy

Valentino Piacentino III

1. Describe the normal flow of blood through the body.

The right atrium of the heart receives blood that has passed through the tissues and given up most of its oxygen. This unoxygenated blood enters the right atrium by two primary vessels, the superior and inferior vena cava. The blood passes from the right atrium into the right ventricle through the tricuspid valve. From the right ventricle the blood is pumped through the pulmonary valve into the pulmonary arteries. The pulmonary arteries flow into the lungs, where the blood becomes oxygenated. Pulmonary veins containing the oxygenated blood pass from the lungs to the left atrium of the heart. Blood then flows from the left atrium into the left ventricle through the bicuspid or mitral valve. Oxygenated blood is pumped from the left ventricle into the aorta through the aortic valve. The aorta branches into many arteries that supply oxygen to all the tissues of the body.

2. Briefly describe the important aspects of the cardiac examination.

- First, ensure one has the proper equipment, including a stethoscope, blood pressure cuff, and pen light.
- Then, visually assess the patient. Is the patient cyanotic; does the patient have edema, shortness of breath, or digital clubbing?
- Next, assess the pulses. Determine the pulse rate; describe the regularity and quality of the pulses. Assess the patient's blood pressure with a stethoscope. Make sure you can auscultate the Korotkoff sounds to accurately measure blood pressure.
- Next, use the stethoscope to assess cardiac sounds on the five anatomical chest landmarks. Are the normal first and second heart sounds heard? Is there abnormal splitting of the heart sounds; are there murmurs? The pen light may be used to closely observe any chest heaving as well as to assess the jugular veins.

3. Describe the origin of the heartbeat and the path of cardiac conduction.

The normal initiation of the heartbeat is from the sinoatrial (SA) node. This specialized area of heart tissue is located in the upper right atrium near the superior vena cava. It is the pacemaker of the heart and normally causes the heart to beat 60 to 80 beats per minute. The SA node produces an electrical stimulus that travels through the atrial tissue to the atrioventricular (AV) node, and then the atria contract. The impulse is delayed briefly at the AV node to allow the atria time to finish contracting before it passes to the bundle of His. This conduction tissue extends down the interventricular septum of the heart as the left and right bundle branches until it reaches the Purkinje fibers. These fibers then transmit the electrical stimulus to the heart muscle and cause ventricular contraction.

4. **What is the average weight of the adult male heart?**

300 grams

5. **What factors may affect heart size?**
   - Body build
   - Age
   - Physical exercise
   - Underlying heart disease

6. **What is the fibrous skeleton of the heart and why is it important?**

The fibrous skeleton of the heart is composed of dense collagen that acts to support the four cardiac valves and to attach the myocardium. This construction of the fibrous skeleton allows for a twisting motion during contraction that imparts efficient contraction and relaxation of the ventricles. The fibrous skeleton also is important as an electrical isolator between the atria and ventricles, allowing conduction only through the AV node in normal individuals. Pathological bypass tracts that allow electrical conduction between the atria and ventricles other than through the AV node can cause life-threatening arrhythmias.

7. **Describe the four layers of heart tissue.**

The four layers of heart tissue (from outer layer inward) are the pericardium (fibrous and visceral), epicardium, myocardium, and endocardium. The pericardium is a saclike structure that contains the heart. The fibrous pericardium is separated from the epicardium by a thin layer of fluid. The epicardium contains the majority of the large coronary arteries before they branch and penetrate the heart muscle. The myocardium is a thick layer of heart muscle cells and is the major contributor to the force generation of the heart. The innermost layer, the endocardium, contains the cardiac conduction tissue and the papillary muscles that tether the mitral and tricuspid valves. The subendocardium is the most vulnerable of the heart structures to a decrease in blood flow (ischemia).

8. **How much fluid is usually present in the pericardial cavity?**

Usually 10 to 30 milliliters of clear serous fluid is present.

9. **What are some functions of the pericardium?**
   - Lubricate the heart
   - Prevent ventricular dilatation
   - Anchor and protect the heart

10. **What is the circumference of the tricuspid valve?**

    11 centimeters

11. **How many cusps are present in the tricuspid valve?**

    Three cusps: the anterior, septal, and posterior

12. **Describe the blood supply to heart muscle.**

    The heart muscle receives oxygen and nutrients through the coronary arteries. The coronary arteries run along the epicardium and then penetrate the muscle to supply the myocardium and endocardium. The two main coronary arteries are the right and left coronaries, and both receive blood from the base of the aorta immediately above the aortic valve. The left coronary artery supplies the interventricular septum and the anterior and lateral left ventricle. The right coronary artery supplies the right ventricle, the posterior left ventricle, and the cardiac conduction system. However, there is some overlap in the parts of the heart the coronary arteries supply, and older individuals can have collateral arteries that connect the right and left coronary arteries.

13. **What procedure is used to visualize the blood supply of the heart?**

    A coronary angiogram is a procedure in which a catheter is inserted into a systemic artery (for example, femoral artery) and passed up the aorta to the origin of the coronary arteries. Radiopaque dye is then injected into the coronary arteries, and a real-time video radiograph is taken to view the distribution and pattern of the coronary arteries. Blockages and occlusions can then be assessed and treated.

14. **What structures lie between the right atrium and right ventricle, and between the left atrium and left ventricle? What separates the ventricles?**

    The right atrium and right ventricle are separated by the right atrioventricular sulcus. The right coronary artery lies within this groove.

    The left atrium and left ventricle are separated by the left atrioventricular sulcus. In this groove lie the circumflex coronary artery (a branch of the left main coronary artery) and the coronary sinus (the main venous drainage vessel of the heart muscle).

    Separating the ventricles on the anterior and posterior surfaces are the anterior and posterior interventricular sulci, respectively. The left anterior descending (LAD) coronary artery and great cardiac vein lie in the anterior interventricular sulcus, and the posterior descending coronary artery is located within the posterior interventricular sulcus.

15. **Which coronary artery supplies the SA node, AV node, and bundle of His?**

    The SA node, AV node, and bundle of His are supplied by the right coronary artery. This is important because occlusion of blood flow in the right coronary artery often causes arrhythmias and possibly bradycardia.

16. **Which coronary artery supplies the bundle branches?**

The bundle branches are supplied by the septal branches of the left anterior descending coronary artery.

17. **What are the branches of the left anterior descending artery?**

- First diagonal
- First septal
- Apical
- Right ventricular
- Second diagonal
- Minor septal

18. **What part of the heart does the circumflex artery supply?**

The left atrium and left ventricle

19. **What are the branches of the circumflex artery?**

- Sinus node artery
- Posterolateral
- Obtuse marginal
- Atrial circumflex

20. **Besides increasing coronary flow can the heart increase oxygen extraction?**

No. The heart extracts the maximal amount of oxygen that passes through the coronary arteries. The heart increases coronary flow to increase oxygen and nutrient delivery.

21. **Where are the proper anatomical landmarks for listening to the four cardiac valves?**

Anatomical landmarks for cardiac valve auscultation

Cardiac Valve	Anatomical Landmarks for Stethoscope Placement
Tricuspid valve	Left fourth and fifth interspaces, parasternal
Pulmonic valve	Left second interspace, parasternal
Mitral valve	Fifth interspace, midclavicular line near point of maximal impact (PMI)
Aortic valve	Right second interspace, parasternal

Data from Bickley L: The Cardiovascular System. In Bickley L: *Guide to Physical Examination and History Taking,* ed 7, pp 277-332, Philadelphia, 1999, Lippincott.

22. How many leaflets does each cardiac valve have?

The aortic, pulmonic, and tricuspid valves have three cusps while the mitral valve has two cusps. The mitral and tricuspid valves are connected to their corresonding ventricles through the chordae tendineae and papillary muscles. The aortic and pulmonic valves are not connected to their ventricles. Remember that the valves open and close because of pressure differences across the valve, not the contraction of the ventricular muscle.

23. Describe the physiology of cardiac murmurs.

Murmurs are sounds caused by myocardial tissue vibration and/or turbulent blood flow. Abrupt changes in blood direction or jets of blood flowing through a narrowing in the circulation produce turbulence. In the case of cardiac valves, abnormalities can cause four classic murmurs. The aortic valve can be stenosed (narrowed) and create a systolic murmur, or the valve may be incompetent, causing blood regurgitation into the left ventricle and a diastolic murmur. The mitral valve can cause a diastolic murmur if it is stenotic, and with an incompetent mitral valve a systolic murmur can occur. Abnormalities with the pulmonic valve will produce murmurs similar to those caused by aortic valve abnormalities, and abnormalities of the tricuspid valve will cause murmurs similar to those caused by mitral valve abnormalities.

Cardiac valve abnormalities and associated murmurs

	Murmur Auscultated in:	
	Systole	Diastole
Aortic valve stenosis	•	
Aortic valve regurgitation		•
Pulmonic valve stenosis	•	
Pulmonic valve regurgitation		•
Mitral valve stenosis		•
Mitral valve regurgitation	•	
Tricuspid valve stenosis		•
Tricuspid valve regurgitation	•	

Data from Bickley L: The Cardiovascular System. In Bickley L: *Guide to Physical Examination and History Taking*, ed 7, pp 277-332, Philadelphia, 1999, Lippincott.

24. Describe the grading of cardiac murmurs.

Grading scale of cardiac murmurs

Grade	Intensity
1/6	Very faint
2/6	Loud and noticeable
3/6	Louder than grade 2
4/6	Louder than grade 3 with associated thrill
5/6	Audible with stethoscope partially above chest wall, with thrill
6/6	Audible with stethoscope barely touching the chest wall

Data from Bickley L: The Cardiovascular System. In Bickley L: *Guide to Physical Examination and History Taking*, ed 7, pp 277-332, Philadelphia, 1999, Lippincott.

25. In the absence of valvular abnormalities, what can cause a systolic murmur?

A systolic murmur in the absence of valvular abnormalities may be caused by a ventricular septal defect. The ventricles (and the atria) of the heart are normally separated by a wall of muscle called the interventricular septum (IVS). In addition to separating the right and left sides of the heart, the IVS contains cardiac conduction tissue. A ventricular septal defect can occur from damage to the muscle tissue of the IVS during a severe MI (myocardial infarction). Because the left ventricle produces a pressure of 120/0 mm Hg and the right ventricle a pressure of 20/7 mm Hg, during systole blood will move from the left ventricle through the hole in the septum to the right ventricle. This is called a left to right shunt and will produce a murmur on auscultation.

26. What do the first (S_1) and second (S_2) heart sounds represent?

S_1 represents the sound of tissue vibration during closure of the mitral and tricuspid valves. The second heart sound (S_2) results from tissue vibrations during closure of the aortic and pulmonic valves. The second heart sound may split (two components may be audible) with inspiration and expiration. Pathological changes in the pulmonary artery pressures can alter the splitting of S_2.

27. Where on the chest wall is the first heart sound (S_1) heard loudest?

At the apex of the heart

28. What is meant by the third heart sound (S_3)?

S_3 is a low-intensity, low-pitch heart sound referred to as a ventricular gallop. S_3 may be normal in young adults and children. However, in individuals over

40 years of age it may represent a noncompliant ventricle in the setting of heart failure. It is best heard in a very quiet environment with the bell of the stethoscope at the left sternal border.

29. What is meant by the fourth heart sound (S₄)?

S_4 is a low-intensity, low-pitch heart sound referred to as an atrial gallop. S_4 is heard before the first heart sound (S_1) and may represent a noncompliant ventricle in the setting of hypertension or a myocardial infarction. S_4 is not heard in patients with atrial fibrillation. It is best heard in a very quiet environment with the bell of the stethoscope over the apex of the left ventricle, and the patient in the left lateral decubitus position.

30. What is coronary ischemia and how can it lead to myocardial infarction?

Coronary ischemia is decreased blood flow to the heart muscle. This can be caused by an occlusion of a coronary artery or a decrease in perfusion pressure to the coronaries. Coronary ischemia will decrease nutrient and oxygen delivery as well as removal of waste products such as carbon dioxide and lactate. Myocardial infarction is death of heart tissue when blood flow is decreased for a prolonged period of time (greater than 40 minutes). Once the tissue has died there is no mechanism for replacement of heart muscle (the heart cannot repair itself). Scar formation may occur and can change the contractility and size of the ventricle.

Key Points

- The heart is composed of four layers of cardiac tissue: the pericardium, endocardium, myocardium, and epicardium.
- Cardiac auscultation is guided by anatomical landmarks on the chest wall.
- The Levine scale grades murmurs according to their intensity or loudness; the scale ranges from grade 1 (barely audible) to grade 6 (murmur heard with the stethoscope barely touching the chest wall).

Internet Resources

Cardiac Anatomy Illustrations:
http://www.ctsnet.org/residents/ctsn/archives/not02.html

Nurse Beat: Cardiac Nursing Electronic Journal:
http://www.cardioconsult.com/Anatomy

Bibliography

Bickley L: The Cardiovascular System. In Bickley L: *Guide to Physical Examination and History Taking*, ed 7, pp 277-332, Philadelphia, 1999, Lippincott.

Braunwald E, Zipes DP, Libby P: *Heart Disease: A Textbook of Cardiovascular Medicine*, ed 6, Philadelphia, 2001, WB Saunders.

Schoen FJ: The Heart. In *Robbins Pathological Basis of Disease*, ed 6, Philadelphia, 1999, WB Saunders.

Chapter 2

Cardiac Physiology

Valentino Piacentino III

1. **What events are taking place during the cardiac cycle?**
   - Electrical activity
   - Atrial, ventricular, and aortic pressure changes
   - Atrial and ventricular volume changes
   - Valvular function
   - Heart sounds

2. **Describe the cardiac cycle.**

   The cardiac cycle is composed of two main segments: systole and diastole. During the beginning of diastolic filling, the ventricles are relaxed, the aortic and pulmonic valves are closed, and the mitral and tricuspid valves are open. Blood passively fills the ventricles and then the atria contract to finish ventricular filling. The end of diastole is triggered by closure of the mitral and tricuspid valves. Now the ventricles begin to contract. This is the beginning of systole. All of the cardiac valves are closed, so this phase is termed the isovolumic period. Once the ventricles generate enough pressure to open up the aortic and pulmonic valves, the valves open and ejection begins. Blood is then pumped into the systemic and pulmonic circulation. When the blood moves more peripheral in the respective circulation, the valves close, the systolic phase of the cardiac cycle ends, and the ventricles begin to relax. Again, all cardiac valves are closed, and this phase is termed isovolumic relaxation and the beginning of diastole. As the pressure drops in the ventricles, the mitral and tricuspid valves open and diastolic filling begins.

3. **How is the first heart sound generated?**
   - Closure of the mitral and tricuspid valves
   - Opening of the aortic and pulmonic valves

4. **How is the second heart sound generated?**

   Closure of the aortic and pulmonic valves

5. **What are normal values for cardiac vital signs, including heart rate (HR), blood pressure (BP), and cardiac output (CO), and how are they measured?**

Normal cardiac hemodynamic values and measurement techniques

	Normal Range	Measurement Technique
Heart rate (HR)	60-80 beats/min	Electrocardiogram, pulse
Arterial blood pressure (ABP)	120/80 mm Hg	Blood pressure cuff; radial, femoral arterial catheter
Pulmonary artery pressure (PAP)	15/7 mm Hg, mean 12 mm Hg	Pulmonary artery catheter
Pulmonary occlusion pressure (PCWP)	4 mm Hg	Pulmonary artery catheter with balloon inflated
Central venous pressure (CVP)	4 mm Hg	Venous catheter in superior vena cava
Cardiac index	2.2-2.8 L/min/m^2	Pulmonary artery catheter with thermodilution capabilities
Systemic vascular resistance (SVR)	900-1300 (dyne-sec)/cm^2	Calculate from mean arterial pressure and cardiac output

Data from Braunwald E, Zipes DP, Libby P: *Heart Disease: A Textbook of Cardiovascular Medicine*, ed 6, Philadelphia, 2001, WB Saunders.

6. **Why are pulmonary pressures less than systemic pressures?**

The right heart pumps blood into the pulmonary circulation, which has a much lower resistance than the systemic circulation. Therefore the pulmonary artery pressure value in a person with normal heart and lung function is 20 to 25% of the blood pressure value in the systemic circulation. Elevation in these pressures can suggest left ventricular failure or primary pulmonary hypertension.

7. **What is the pulmonary wedge pressure and what does it represent?**

The pulmonary wedge pressure (also known as pulmonary capillary wedge pressure [PCWP]) is an estimate of the filling pressure of the left ventricle. It is measured with a pulmonary artery catheter (PAC), which is inserted through a systemic vein (jugular, femoral, or subclavian) and advanced through the right ventricle into the pulmonary artery. The pulmonary wedge pressure can be used to assess the volume status and the contractility of the left ventricle. Volume overload and/or heart failure can elevate the pulmonary wedge pressure.

8. **Describe systolic and diastolic blood pressure.**

    The systolic blood pressure is the maximum pressure in the large arteries of the systemic circulation during ventricular ejection; the diastolic blood pressure is the lowest blood pressure during the cardiac cycle.

9. **When during the cardiac cycle is coronary blood flow the greatest and why?**

    Unlike other organs, blood flow to the heart muscle itself through the coronaries is highest during diastole. During systole the heart muscle is contracting and the pressure in the tissue surrounding the coronaries is high, decreasing blood flow. During diastole the heart muscle is relaxing and the coronaries have their greatest flow. This is a very important concept to remember because if diastolic blood pressure is too low it can decrease coronary blood flow and cause ischemia. Also, high heart rates can decrease the time of diastole and decrease coronary blood flow.

10. **Describe the baroreceptors and their associated reflex.**

    The baroreceptors are a group of specialized cells located in the aortic arch and carotid bodies that sense the arterial blood pressure (ABP). As blood pressure rises, they stretch and send impulses to the brainstem (medulla). A decrease in blood pressure has the opposite effect. These receptors allow the body to regulate sympathetic and parasympathetic neural outflow to the heart and blood vessels as a means of controlling blood pressure. This feedback circuit is termed the baroreceptor reflex.

11. **What are the two major factors that determine the mean blood pressure?**

    Blood pressure is influenced by two main physiological factors: the cardiac output of the heart and the systemic vascular resistance (SVR) of the systemic circulation.

12. **What determines cardiac output?**

    Cardiac output can be calculated as the product of heart rate and stroke volume. Factors that determine the cardiac output are heart rate, heart rhythm, preload, afterload, and contractility. Heart rate and heart rhythm primarily regulate the frequency of heartbeats and the degree of coordination of each contraction. Preload, afterload, and contractility determine the stroke volume (the amount of blood ejected with each heartbeat). Remember that at high heart rates cardiac filling may be impaired and stroke volume will decrease.

Equations used in evaluating cardiac hemodynamics

Parameter (Abbreviation)	Formula
Mean arterial pressure (MAP)	$MAP = CO \times TPR(SVR)$
Cardiac output (CO)	$CO = SV \times HR$
Stroke volume (SV)	$SV = EDV - ESV$
Ejection fraction (EF)	$EF = \dfrac{SV}{EDV}$
Heart rate (HR)	
Systemic vascular resistance (SVR)	$SVR = 80 \times \dfrac{(MAP - CVP)}{CO}$
Pulmonary vascular resistance (PVR)	$PVR = 80 \times \dfrac{(MPAP - PCWP)}{CO}$

SVR is also known as total peripheral resistance (TPR).
Data from Braunwald E, Zipes DP, Libby P: *Heart Disease: A Textbook of Cardiovascular Medicine*, ed 6, Philadelphia, 2001, WB Saunders.

13. Describe cardiac preload and afterload.

Preload describes how much blood is in the heart before each heartbeat. In the case of the left ventricle it can be estimated via the pulmonary wedge pressure. Again, in a normal patient increasing the preload increases the cardiac output. This is described as the Starling mechanism of the heart. Afterload can be described as the pressure the heart has to work against to open the aortic (left ventricle) or pulmonic (right ventricle) valve to eject blood into the lungs or systemic circulation. A good measure of afterload is the arterial blood pressure. A decrease in afterload ("unloading the ventricle") can increase cardiac output in end-stage heart failure patients.

14. What is systemic vascular resistance (SVR)?

SVR is a measure of the resistance to blood flow offered by the systemic arterial bed. It is controlled at the arteriole and capillary levels by neural input and circulating hormones. Pathological conditions, such as shock and congestive heart failure, can alter SVR. Also vasodilator agents (nitrates) can decrease SVR and vasoconstrictors (vasopressin, norepinephrine, neosynephrine) can increase SVR. An increase in SVR can help increase blood pressure to the brain and heart but also makes the heart work harder.

15. What is stroke volume?

Stroke volume is the volume of blood ejected by the ventricle in a single contraction.

16. What is ejection fraction?

The percentage of the total ventricular volume ejected during each contraction is the ejection fraction.

17. What is the normal ejection fraction?

55% to 65%

18. What is normal oxygen consumption?

200 to 250 milliliters per minute

19. What are the determinants of oxygen consumption?

• Cardiac output
• Hemoglobin levels
• Partial pressure of oxygen
• Arterial oxygen saturation

20. What is cardiac contractility?

Think of contractility (or the inotropic state) as the intrinsic ability of the heart muscle itself to pump blood (independent of preload and afterload). When contractility increases, cardiac output increases (similar to what happens during exercise). Patients with hyperthyroidism and pheochromocytomas usually have increased contractility while patients with heart failure or myocardial infarctions typically have decreased contractility.

21. What pharmacological agents can help a failing ventricle with decreased contractility?

Inotropic agents (such as dobutamine, epinephrine, and milrinone) increase the ability of the heart to pump blood (contractility). They work at the cellular level, increasing the force that each individual heart muscle cell can generate. Thus, inotropic agents increase the contractility of the heart. This can increase cardiac output and blood pressure. To review, the factors that influence cardiac output are heart rate, heart rhythm, preload, afterload, and contractility.

22. How can you distinguish between left and right ventricular failure?

High pulmonary wedge pressures, decreased exercise capacity, and pulmonary congestion characterize left ventricular failure. Isolated right ventricular failure is characterized by jugular venous distention (JVD), hepatomegaly (large liver), and peripheral edema. It is important to remember that the main cause of right ventricular failure is left ventricular failure. Thus patients with severe left ventricular failure can develop JVD, hepatomegaly and peripheral edema.

23. Describes the features of the ECG (electrocardiogram).

The beginning of the electrocardiogram is the P wave, which represents the activation of the atrium by the sinoatrial (SA) node. This is followed by a short pause and then the **QRS** complex. This part of the waveform occurs during the beginning of electrical activation of the right and left ventricles. After the QRS complex is the T wave. The T wave represents the end of the electrical activation of the ventricle. In normal sinus rhythm the T wave is followed by the P wave of the next heartbeat, and the subsequent QRS complex and T wave. Irregularities in the heartbeat, or dysrhythmias, can be detected via the electrocardiogram.

24. What are normal values for the components of the ECG?

The **PR interval** (the time from the beginning of the P wave to the beginning of the QRS complex) should be 120 to 200 milliseconds. The **QRS complex** should be no longer than 100 milliseconds, and the **QT interval** (from the beginning of the QRS complex to the end of the T wave) should be less than 440 milliseconds when corrected for heart rate. The corrected QT interval is $QT/\sqrt{R} - R$. The upper limit of the corrected QT interval is 0.42 second.

25. What does the term "reflex-tachycardia" mean?

When a pharmacological agent that decreases SVR (for example, nitrates, vasodilators) is administered, blood pressure may decrease to the point that the baroreceptor reflex increases the heart rate to compensate and increase cardiac output. Sometimes beta-blockers are given along with these agents to eliminate the reflex-tachycardia.

26. What is ventricular fibrillation (VFib) and is it a life-threatening dysrhythmia?

Ventricular fibrillation is an unorganized, chaotic rhythm of the heart ventricle that does not allow coordinated contraction of the ventricle and normal ejection of blood. Yes, this rhythm is life-threatening because it will not generate blood pressure, which results in brain and heart ischemia. Immediate treatment includes cardiopulmonary resuscitation and defibrillation. Pharmacological agents used to treat VFib include lidocaine and amiodarone.

27. What is the function of a defibrillator?

A defibrillator is a device that can give a short, powerful burst of electrical energy to a person sustaining a life-threatening cardiac arrhythmia. When a short burst of electrical energy is delivered to the heart during an arrhythmia (atrial fibrillation, ventricular tachycardia and fibrillation), the heart rhythm may be able to "reset" (defibrillate) and the SA node can regain control of the heartbeat.

28. **What is an automatic internal cardiac defibrillator (AICD)?**

AICDs are devices implanted in patients who have a history of arrhythmias and/or are at risk for irregular, life-threatening heart rhythms. It is implanted under the skin, similar to a pacemaker, and can detect irregular heart rhythms and deliver an electrical shock to the heart to help return the heart to a normal rhythm. The AICD is similar to the defibrillator used in an intensive care unit (ICU). The difference is that the implanted defibrillator, unlike the ICU defibrillator, can detect irregular heartbeats. Therefore individuals working in the ICU need to be able to recognize irregular heart rhythms.

29. **Why is regulation of serum potassium (K^+) concentration important with regard to the cardiac conduction system?**

Potassium is the major electrolyte the heart uses to control the duration of the heartbeat, which can be measured with the ECG. Normal K concentration in a blood sample is 3.5 to 5.3 millimoles per liter and is closely regulated in the body. An increase in the K concentration (hyperkalemia) can slow the heart rate and cause changes in the ECG and arrhythmias, such as peaked T waves, ST depression, and subsequent slow heart rate (bradycardia). A decrease in serum K concentration (hypokalemia) can also cause changes in the electrocardiogram and arrhythmias, such as decreased T wave amplitude, flattened ST segment, and ventricular ectopy (an abnormal heartbeat arising from a location in the heart other than the SA node). Also, in addition to patients undergoing cardiac procedures, it is very important to watch the K concentration in patients with abnormal kidney function, patients with diabetes mellitus, and patients receiving diuretics.

30. **Why is it important to monitor serum calcium (Ca^{++}) concentration in the cardiac patient?**

The level of Ca^{++}, along with K^+, is highly regulated inside heart muscle. It is Ca^{++} that causes the heart muscle to generate force. Decreases in Ca^{++} levels can decrease the inotropic state (contractility) of the heart and contribute to poor cardiac output. Inotropic agents, such as dobutamine, cause an increase in Ca^{++} levels in the heart muscle, resulting in greater heart contractility.

 ## Key Points

- Coronary flow is greatest during diastole.
- Blood pressure is determined by cardiac output and systemic vascular resistance.
- The concepts of preload and afterload are important in the understanding of cardiac physiology. Preload is the amount of blood in the heart after each heartbeat. Afterload is the pressure the heart has to work against to open the aortic valve or pulmonic valve to eject blood into the lungs or the systemic circulation.

Internet Resources

Cardiovascular Physiology Concepts:
http://www.oucom.ohiou.edu/CVPhysiology

The Gross Physiology of the Cardiovascular System:
http://cardiovascular.cx

Bibliography

Braunwald E, Zipes DP, Libby P: *Heart Disease: A Textbook of Cardiovascular Medicine*, ed 6, Philadelphia, 2001, WB Saunders.

Hypertension

Sandra Davis

1. How is blood pressure (BP) classified?

According to the guidelines of JNC VII (*The Seventh Report of the Joint National Committee on Prevention, Detection, Evaluation, and Treatment of High Blood Pressure*), there are four classifications for blood pressure.

Classification of blood pressure

Blood Pressure Classification	Systolic Blood Pressure (SBP), mm Hg	Diastolic Blood Pressure (DBP), mm Hg
Normal	<120	<80
Pre-hypertension	120-139	80-89
Stage I hypertension	140-159	90-99
Stage II hypertension	≥160	≥100

From U.S. Department of Health and Human Services, National Institutes of Health, National Heart, Lung, and Blood Institute: *The seventh report of the joint national committee on prevention, detection, evaluation, and treatment of high blood pressure*, NIH publication number 03-5233, 2003.

2. What is the proper technique for taking a blood pressure measurement?

When taking a blood pressure measurement, it is important to use a device that has been properly calibrated. The patient should be calm and should have been seated in a chair for at least 5 minutes. Ideally the patient should not have ingested tea or coffee 1 hour before blood pressure measurement, and the patient should not have smoked cigarettes within 15 minutes of blood pressure measurement. The patient's arm should be supported at heart level. Improper cuff size can lead to falsely elevated or reduced blood pressure readings. The bladder cuff should encircle at least 80% of the arm. At least two measurements should be taken. Verification should be established by also taking a BP measurement in the contralateral arm.

A greater than 10 mm Hg discrepancy in blood pressure readings from arm to arm may indicate subclavian disease. The presence of subclavian disease may preclude the use of the internal thoracic artery for coronary artery bypass grafting. Both verbal and written results of the blood pressure reading should be conveyed to the patient.

3. **What is the relationship between hypertension (HTN) and cardiovascular disease (CVD)?**

According to JNC VII, the relationship between hypertension and CVD is continuous, consistent, and independent of other risk factors for CVD. Higher BP results in a greater chance of heart attack, heart failure, stroke, and kidney disease. Starting at a BP of 115/75 mm Hg, the risk of CVD doubles with each incremental increase of 20/10 mm Hg.

4. **What is the pathophysiology of hypertension?**

The exact mechanism of hypertension is unclear, but it is believed to be multifactorial. Genetic, environmental, and lifestyle influences all work in concert to produce HTN. Proposed physiologic mechanisms of primary HTN include:
  - Abnormalities within the autonomic nervous system:
    - Insensitivity of the baroreceptor reflex or sympathetic hyperactivity
  - Abnormalities within the renin-angiotensin system:
    - Decreased BP = increased renin levels = increased angiotensin I levels → angiotensin II production
  - Abnormalities in vascular autoregulation:
    - Abnormal nitric oxide levels
  - Abnormalities in intravascular fluid volume:
    - Decreased volume = decreased venous return = decreased cardiac output (CO) + increased renal blood flow = aldosterone stimulation = sodium and water retention = increased BP

5. **What are the different types of hypertension?**
  - Primary hypertension
  - Secondary hypertension
  - Isolated systolic hypertension
  - Malignant hypertension
  - Accelerated-malignant hypertension
  - White-coat hypertension

6. **What is primary hypertension?**

Primary HTN is also known as essential HTN and was once considered to be idiopathic. Primary HTN occurs in 95% of hypertension cases, and the exact cause is thought to be multifactorial. It is believed that both genetic and environmental factors play a role. The onset is usually between the ages of 25 and 55 years, and there is usually a positive family history.

7. **What is secondary hypertension?**

Secondary HTN represents 5% of the cases of HTN and can be attributed to specific causes. Secondary HTN causes include:
- Coarctation of the aorta
- Cushing's syndrome
- Pheochromocytoma
- Primary aldosteronism
- Renal disease
- Renal vascular disease
- Increased intracranial pressure (ICP)
- Acute pancreatitis
- Thyrotoxicosis
- Sleep apnea
- Drug-induced secondary HTN:
  - Amphetamines
  - Cocaine
  - Oral contraceptives
  - Estrogen
  - Corticosteriods
  - Licorice
  - Thyroid hormone
  - Immunosuppressives

8. **What is isolated systolic hypertension?**

Isolated systolic HTN is common with aging and may account for up to 65% to 75% of HTN in the elderly.

9. **What is malignant hypertension?**

Malignant HTN is a sustained HTN that requires immediate therapy. Patients usually have symptoms of headache, blurred or decreased vision, chest pain, and/or confusion. In addition they have new or progressive end-organ damage, resulting in encephalopathy, nephropathy, and papilledema. The damage results in renal failure, heart failure, and myocardial infarction (MI) if left untreated.

10. **What is accelerated hypertension?**

Accelerated hypertension is a milder form of malignant hypertension in which the patient may be symptomatic but encephalopathy, nephropathy, and papilledema are not present.

11. **What is white coat hypertension?**

White-coat hypertension, also known as isolated clinical hypertension, refers to a blood pressure reading that is normal when taken outside of the hospital or provider office setting but is consistently high when taken in the office or hospital setting. Ambulatory blood pressure monitoring (ABPM) is useful for identifying patients with white-coat hypertension.

12. What are the risk factors for primary hypertension?

- Tobacco use
- High sodium diet
- Low dietary intake of potassium, calcium, and magnesium
- Diet high in saturated fats
- Obesity
- Sedentary lifestyle
- Stress
- Caffeine ingestion
- Glucose intolerance
- Family history
- Advancing age
- Gender (men <50 years, women >50 years)
- Heavy alcohol intake
- African-American race

13. What are the clinical manifestations of hypertension?

HTN is known as the silent killer because it usually does not produce symptoms. Therefore it often goes undetected while it renders harmful effects on several target organs or end organs within the body.

14. What organs are known as target organs (end organs), and how is hypertension manifested within those organs?

Organ	Manifestations
Heart	Heart failure
	Coronary artery disease
	Left ventricular dysfunction
	Left ventricular hypertrophy
Brain	Transient ischemic attack
	Cerebrovascular accident (CVA)
	Headache
Kidneys	Renal insufficiency
	Proteinuria
	Microalbuminuria
Eyes	Retinopathy

15. When obtaining a thorough patient history for a patient with hypertension or suspected hypertension, what important questions should be included?

A thorough patient history should emphasize:
- Family history of HTN
- Known duration and levels of elevated BP

- History of tobacco use, dietary habits, alcohol intake, weight gain, daily schedule, leisure activities, hobbies, physical activities, and exercise
- Side effects, if any, of previous antihypertensives
- Signs and symptoms that are suggestive of secondary HTN
- Psychosocial and environmental conditions including coping mechanisms and support systems

16. What is orthostatic or postural hypotension?

Orthostatic hypotension is a drop in BP when an upright posture is assumed. It occurs more frequently in older patients who have systolic hypertension or diabetes and in patients taking diuretics, venodilators, and some psychotropic drugs.

17. What are the symptoms of orthostatic hypotension?

There may be no symptoms at all or the following symptoms: light-headedness, dizziness, weakness, unsteadiness, visual blurring, presyncope, or syncope.

18. What is the proper technique for taking orthostatic blood pressure measurements?

There are several techniques for taking orthostatic blood pressures. One technique may include:
- Measuring blood pressure and pulse rate after 5 minutes of lying supine
- Repeating the measurement immediately upon standing, and again after 1 to 3 minutes of continued standing
- Substituting the sitting position for the standing position if the patient is not able to stand or if it is unsafe for the patient to stand

A decrease in the systolic blood pressure of 20 mm Hg or more, a decrease in the diastolic blood pressure of 10 mm Hg or more, or an increase in the pulse rate of 20 beats per minute or more at any point would be indicative of orthostasis.

19. What is the rationale for the use of ambulatory blood pressure monitoring (ABPM)?

On the basis of various clinical trials, it is believed that target-organ or end-organ damage associated with hypertension is more closely related to APBM than clinical or casual blood pressure measurements. Ambulatory blood pressure monitors are currently lightweight, easy to wear, programmable, computer-interactive, and accurate. Interpretation of ABPM should include mean daytime, nighttime (sleep), and 24-hour measurements in conjunction with a diary of medications and the time of their administration.

20. What are the routine tests that are recommended before initiating antihypertensive therapy?

- Serum potassium level
- Hemoglobin and hematocrit levels

- Fasting blood glucose value
- Creatinine clearance or glomerular filtration rate (GFR)
- Fasting lipid profile
- Electrocardiogram (ECG)
- Urinalysis

21. What must a physical examination for hypertension or suspected hypertension include?

- Proper blood pressure measurement:
  - Including verification in the contralateral arm
- Eye examination:
  - Including fundoscopic examination
- Height, weight, waist circumference:
  - Calculation of the body mass index (BMI)
- Auscultation for bruits:
  - Carotid
  - Abdominal
  - Renal
  - Femoral
- Palpation of the thyroid gland
- Examination of the heart
- Examination of the lungs
- Abdominal exam
- Lower extremity examination
- Neurological examination

22. How is hypertension managed?

JNC VII has established guidelines for the management of hypertension that are based on the finding and results of large-scale randomized clinical trials.

23. What are lifestyle modifications?

Lifestyle modifications are the adaptation of healthy behaviors that have been shown to lower blood pressure. They are:
- Smoking cessation
- Weight reduction in those patients who are overweight or obese:
  - Maintain a BMI of 18.5 to 24.9 kg/m^2
- Adoption of the Dietary Approaches to Stop Hypertension (DASH) eating plan:
  - Eat fruits, vegetables, low-fat dairy products, and foods with reduced saturated and total fat
- Increased physical activity:
  - Engage in regular aerobic physical activity at least 30 minutes per day three or more times per week
- Moderation of alcohol consumption:
  - No more than two drinks per day in most men and no more than one drink per day in most women, depending on individual weight (drink = 1 oz or 30 ml of ethanol, 24 oz of beer, 10 oz of wine, or 3 oz of 80-proof whiskey)

Guidelines for the management of hypertension from JNC VII

BP Classification	SBP, mm Hg	DBP, mm Hg	Lifestyle Modification	Initial Drug Therapy without Compelling Indications	Initial Drug Therapy with Compelling Indications
Normal	<120	<80	Assess and teach*	Hypertensive drug therapy not indicated	Use drugs for compelling indications
Pre-hypertension	120-139	80-89	Yes	Hypertensive drug therapy not indicated	Use drugs for compelling indications
Stage I hypertension	140-159	90-99	Yes	Thiazide diuretics for most; ACEI, ARB, BB, CCB, or combination may be considered	Use drugs for compelling indications; use other antihypertensive drugs (diuretics, ACEI, ARB, BB, CCB) as needed[†]
Stage II hypertension	≥160	≥100	Yes	Two-drug combination for most (usually thiazide-type diuretic and ACEI, ARB, BB, or CCB)[‡]	Use drugs for compelling indications; use other antihypertensive drugs (diuretics, ACEI, ARB, BB, CCB) as needed[†]

From U.S. Department of Health and Human Services, National Institutes of Health, National Heart, Lung, and Blood Institute: *The seventh report of the joint national committee on prevention, detection, evaluation, and treatment of high blood pressure*, NIH publication number 03-5233, 2003.

SBP, systolic blood pressure; *DBP*, diastolic blood pressure; *ACEI*, angiotensin converting enzyme (ACE) inhibitor (ACEI); *ARB*, angiotensin receptor blocker; *BB*, beta-blocker; *CCB*, calcium channel blocker.

*Treatment is determined by the highest BP category.

[†]Treat patients with chronic renal disease or diabetes to goal BP <130/80 mm Hg.

[‡]Initial combination therapy should be used with caution in patients at risk for orthostatic hypotension.

24. **What are compelling indications when referring to management of hypertension?**

Compelling indications are certain comorbidities that the hypertensive patient may have that require particular antihypertensive drug classes. The comorbid conditions include:
- Ischemic heart disease:
  - First drug of choice is usually a beta-blocker if there are no contraindications to its use
- Heart failure:
  - Asymptomatic patients with demonstrable ventricular dysfunction:
    - Angiotensin-converting enzyme (ACE) inhibitors and beta-blockers
  - Symptomatic ventricular dysfunction or end-stage heart disease:
    - ACE inhibitors, beta-blockers, angiotensin-receptor blockers, aldosterone blockers, and loop diuretics
- Diabetes and hypertension:
  - Combinations of two or more drugs usually needed to achieve the target goal of <130/80 mm Hg (thiazide diuretics, beta-blockers, ACE inhibitors, calcium channel blockers)
- Chronic kidney disease:
  - ACE inhibitors and angiotensin-receptor blockers
- Cerebrovascular disease:
  - ACE inhibitors and diuretics

25. **What are the major classes of drugs that are used to treat HTN?**

Medications used to treat HTN include the following:
- Thiazide diuretics
- Loop diuretics
- Potassium-sparing diuretics
- Aldosterone receptor blockers
- Beta-blockers
- Combined alpha- and beta-blockers
- ACE inhibitors
- Angiotensin II receptor blockers
- Calcium channel blockers
- Alpha-blockers
- Central alpha agonists
- Vasodilators
- Combination-type drugs
  - ACE inhibitors and calcium channel blockers
  - ACE inhibitors and diuretics
  - Aldosterone receptor blockers and diuretics
  - Beta-blockers and diuretics
  - Centrally acting drugs and diuretics

26. **When is the usual follow-up visit for a patient started on antihypertensive medication?**

Patients should normally return to the provider's office for a follow-up visit and possibly adjustment of their medication on a monthly basis until the BP goal is reached. It has been found that most people with hypertension will require two or more antihypertensive medications to achieve their BP goal. Patients with stage 2 HTN or with comorbid conditions may require more frequent visits. The need for certain laboratory tests may also require more frequent visits. Once the BP goal has been reached, follow-up visits may be at 3- to 6-month intervals.

27. **What is the dysmetabolic syndrome?**

Dysmetabolic syndrome is the presence of three or more of the following conditions:
  - Abdominal obesity:
    - Waist circumference >40 inches in men or >35 inches in women
  - Glucose intolerance:
    - Fasting glucose level ≥110 mg/dl
  - HTN:
    - BP reading ≥130/85 mm Hg
  - High triglyceride levels:
    - ≥150 mg/dl
  - Low HDL levels:
    - <40 mg/dl in men or <50 mg/dl in women

It is believed that those with the dysmetabolic syndrome are at a greater risk of having a myocardial infarction.

28. **What is the difference between hypertensive emergency and hypertensive urgency?**

Both hypertensive emergencies and urgencies are forms of hypertensive crises. In both conditions patients have marked BP elevations. Both situations may produce widespread symptoms, or the patient may be relatively asymptomatic until end-organ damage occurs. Patients with hypertensive emergencies must be treated immediately. This includes hospitalization and treatment with parental antihypertensive agents. With a hypertensive urgency, patients do not necessarily require hospitalization, but they should receive immediate combination oral antihypertensive therapy. In addition, they should be carefully monitored for hypertensive-induced heart or kidney damage and identifiable causes of hypertension.

29. **What is the BP goal while treating a patient with a hypertensive crisis?**

The goal is to reduce the blood pressure slowly. Over a 2- to 6-hour time period, the blood pressure should be reduced to 160/100 mm Hg. Excessive blood pressure reduction can lead to a compromise of the cerebral perfusion, which in turn can precipitate ischemic events in patients with altered cerebral autoregulation.

30. What are the parenteral antihypertensives that are used in treatment of hypertensive emergencies?

- Sodium nitroprusside (Nipride)
- Nitroglycerin
- Diazoxide (Hyperstat)
- Fenoldopam
- Hydralazine
- Enalapril (Vasotec)
- Nicardipine (Cardene)
- Esmolol (Brevibloc)
- Phentolamine (Regitine)
- Labetalol (Normodyne, Trandate)

Key Points

- Isolated systolic hypertension is common in the elderly.
- Types of hypertension include: primary, secondary, isolated systolic, malignant, accelerated malignant, and white coat.
- Pre-hypertension is defined as a blood pressure of 120-139/80-89 mm Hg.

Internet Resources

National Heart, Lung, and Blood Institute:
http://www.nhlbi.nih.gov/guidelines/hypertension

Doctor's Guide: Personal Edition: Hypertension:
http://www.ash-us.org
http://www.about-hypertension.com

Bibliography

Barkley TW, Myers CM: *Practice guidelines for acute care nurse practitioners*, Philadelphia, 2001, WB Saunders.

McGrath BM: Ambulatory blood pressure monitoring, *Med J Austr* 176(17): 588-592, 2002.

Tierney LM, McPhee SJ, Papadakis MK: *Current medical diagnosis and treatment*, New York, 2001, McGraw-Hill.

U.S. Department of Health and Human Services, National Institutes of Health, National Heart, Lung, and Blood Institute: *The seventh report of the joint national committee on prevention, detection, evaluation, and treatment of high blood pressure*, NIH publication number 03-5233, 2003.

Dyslipidemia

Kimberly Ann Devine

1. What are the current American College of Cardiology/American Heart Association (ACC/AHA) recommendations in the management of dyslipidemia?

Current ACC/AHA recommendations in the management of dyslipidemia

Risk	Institute Drug Therapy if LDL Greater Than:	Goal LDL
LOW RISK with <2 of the following: Smoker Hypertensive Positive family history Male >45 years old Female >55 years old (HDL >35 cancels 1 positive risk factor)	190	<160
HIGH RISK with ≥2 of the following: Smoker Hypertensive Positive family history Male >45 years old Female >55 years old (HDL >35 cancels 1 positive risk factor)	160	<130
Known coronary artery disease, diabetic, PVD, carotid disease, AAA	130	<100

Data from 2002 ACC/AHA UA/NSTEMI Guideline Update: available at www.acc.org, 2002.

2. **How is low-density lipoprotein cholesterol (LDL-C) calculated?**

LDL cholesterol is calculated by using the Friedewald formula:

LDL cholesterol (mg/dl) = total cholesterol −

HDL cholesterol − (triglyceride/5)

This formula is not accurate if the triglyceride level is greater than 400 or if the patient is homozygous for apo E_2.

3. **What is the importance of having elevated high-density lipoprotein cholesterol (HDL-C) and reduced low-density lipoprotein cholesterol (LDL-C) levels?**

HDL is known as the good cholesterol and LDL is known as the bad cholesterol. Having high good cholesterol levels and low bad cholesterol levels greatly reduces the chances of sustaining a major adverse cardiac event.

4. **With adequate control of hyperlipidemia, is there a reduction in the incidence of myocardial infarction?**

Yes. In multiple studies, statin therapy (especially in combination with a balanced diet and regular exercise) has been proven to decrease the risk of heart attack and stroke, lessen the need for heart surgery and angioplasty, and reduce the risk of death significantly. It has been estimated that for every 1% decrease in LDL cholesterol and every 1% increase in HDL cholesterol, the risk of adverse cardiovascular events falls by 2% and 3%, respectively.

5. **Name the common causes of primary dyslipidemia.**

- Hypercholesterolemia
- Heterozygous familial hypercholesterolemia
- Homozygous familial hypercholesterolemia
- Familial defective apo B-100
- Polygenic hypercholesterolemia
- Disorders of HDL metabolism
- Familial hypoalphalipoproteinemia
- Familial apo A-I/C-III deficiency
- Tangier disease
- Fish eye disease
- Primary combined hyperlipidemia
- Familial dysbetalipoproteinemia
- Primary hypertriglyceridemia
- Familial hypertriglyceridemia
- Familial hyperchylomicronemia
- Lipoprotein lipase deficiency
- Apolipoprotein C-III deficiency

6. Name the common causes of secondary dyslipidemia.

- Elevated LDL-C levels
- Hypothyroidism
- Nephrotic syndrome
- Anorexia nervosa
- Chronic liver disease
- Dysglobulinemia
- Cholestasis
- Elevated triglyceride levels
- Alcohol abuse
- Diabetes mellitus
- Pregnancy
- Chronic renal failure
- Beta-blocker therapy
- Diuretics
- Exogenous estrogens
- Cushing's syndrome
- Oral contraceptives
- Low HDL-C levels
- Physical inactivity
- Smoking
- Obesity
- Hypertriglyceridemia

7. What classifications of lipid-lowering medications are available?

- Bile acid sequestrants (resins):
  - Cholestyramine
  - Colestipol
  - Colesevelam
  - Nicotinic acid
  - Niacin
  - Niaspan
- HMG-CoA reductase inhibitors:
  - Atorvastatin
  - Fluvastatin
  - Lovastatin
  - Pravastatin
  - Simvastatin
- Fibric acid derivatives:
  - Clofibrate
  - Gemfibrozil
  - Fenofibrate
  - Zetia

8. **What pharmacological options are available in the management of dyslipidemia?**

Pharmacological options for management of dyslipidemia

Drug	Initial Dose	Maintenance Dose	Route	Frequency
Gemfibrozil (Lopid)		300-600 mg	PO	b.i.d.
Lovastatin (Mevacor)	20 mg/day	20-80 mg/day	PO	daily or b.i.d.
Niacin (vitamin B$_3$)		0.5-2.0 g	PO	every day
Pravastatin (Pravachol)	10-20 mg/day	10-40 mg/day	PO	daily at bedtime
Cholestyramine (Questran)	4 g	4-8 g	PO	b.i.d.
Simvastatin (Zocor)	10-20 mg/day	10-40 mg	PO	daily at bedtime
Atorvastatin (Lipitor)	10 mg	10-40 mg	PO	daily at bedtime
Fluvastatin (Lescol)	20 mg	20-80 mg	PO	daily at bedtime
Colesevlam (Welchol)	3 tablets	3 tablets	PO	b.i.d. with meals
	625-mg tablets	6 tablets	PO	daily with meals
Advicor (Niaspan/Lovastatin)	500/20 mg	500/20 mg, 500/40 mg, or 1000/20 mg	PO	daily at bedtime
Rosuvastatin (Crestor)	10 mg/day	5-40 mg/day	PO	daily at bedtime

Data from 2002 ACC/AHA UA/NSTEMI Guideline Update: available at www.acc.org, 2002.

9. **How do bile acid sequestrants (resins) reduce cholesterol?**

Bile acids are synthesized from cholesterol in the liver and are reabsorbed in the small intestine. The resins bind with the bile acids and prevent their reabsorption. As a result, circulating cholesterol levels are reduced.

10. **How do nicotinic acids reduce cholesterol?**

Nicotinic acid is a B vitamin (niacin) that has been found to have lipid-regulating effects at higher doses. It decreases the hepatic synthesis and release of very-low-density lipoprotein (VLDL). Nicotinic acids decrease the plasma levels of free fatty acids, decrease the hepatic production of triglycerides, decrease LDL cholesterol and triglyceride levels, and increase HDL cholesterol levels. There is also some belief that nicotinic acids may inhibit the synthesis of cholesterol within the liver.

11. **How do HMG-CoA reductase inhibitors (statins) decrease cholesterol levels?**

Statin therapy partially inhibits the HMG-CoA reductase enzyme within the liver. Because of the reduction in intracellular cholesterol levels within the liver, there is an upregulation of receptors and enhanced clearance of lipoproteins containing apo B and apo E. As a result there is a reduction in the LDL cholesterol level.

12. **What lab work should be completed before the initiation of statin therapy?**
   - Lipid and lipoprotein profiles
   - Alanine transferase (ALT) levels
   - Aspartate transferase (AST) levels

13. **What are the serious adverse side effects of statin therapy?**
   - Myalgias
   - Rhabdomyolysis

   Although extremely rare, if a patient's symptoms include these side effects, statin therapy should be discontinued and the patient should be referred to a physician for immediate treatment.

14. **When should statin therapy be discontinued?**

   Statin therapy should be continued indefinitely unless the patient's medical condition warrants discontinuation:
   - Transaminase levels >3 times the upper limit of normal
   - Myalgias
   - Myositis
   - Rhabdomyolysis

15. **What medications, when administered with statin therapy, will place the patient at higher risk for myopathies?**
   - Fibrates (especially gemfibrozil)
   - Nicotinic acid (rare)
   - Cyclosporine
   - Azole antifungals
   - Itraconazole
   - Ketoconazole
   - Macrolide antibiotics
   - Erythromycin
   - Clarithromycin
   - HIV protease inhibitors
   - Nefazodone (antidepressant)
   - Verapamil
   - Amiodarone
   - Alcohol abuse

Key Points

- The following laboratory studies should be conducted before the initiation of statin therapy:
  - Lipid and lipoprotein profiles
  - Alanine transferase (ALT) levels
  - Aspartate transferase (AST) levels
- The target LDL cholesterol in a person with no known risk factors is 160.
- The groups of medications used to treat dyslipidemia are:
  - Bile acid sequestrants
  - Fibric acid derivatives
  - HMG-CoA reductase inhibitors
  - Nicotinic acid

Internet Resources

Lipidhealth: Dyslipidemia Resources:
http://www.dyslipidemia.org

Lipids Online: Educational Resources in Atherosclerosis:
http://www.lipidsonline.org

Bibliography

2002 ACC/AHA UA/NSTEMI Guideline Update: available at www.acc.org, 2002.

Braunwald E: *Heart Disease: A Textbook of Cardiovascular Medicine*, ed 5, Philadelphia, 1997, WB Saunders.

Califf RM: *ACS Essentials*, Mich, 2003, Physician Press.

Cor Therapeutics and Key Pharmaceuticals: www.integrilin.com, 2000.

Eli-Lilly: www.reopro.com, 2000.

Gawlinski A, Hamwi D: *Acute Care Nurse Practitioner: Clinical Curriculum and Certification Review*, Philadelphia, 1999, WB Saunders.

Grimes C: Presentation at ACC, Beamont University Hospital, March 2003.

Hazinski MF, Cummins RO, Field JM: *Handbook of Emergency Cardiovascular Care*, Tex, 2000, American Heart Association.

Isselbacher KJ, Braunwald E, Wilson JD, Martin JB, Fauci AS, Kasper DL: *Harrison's Principles of Internal Medicine*, ed 15, New York, 2001, McGraw-Hill.

Marso SP, Griffin BP, Topol EJ: *Manual of Cardiovascular Medicine*, Philadelphia, 2000, Lippincott Williams & Wilkins.

Merck: www.aggrastat.com, 2003.

Coronary Artery Disease

Kimberly Ann Devine

1. What are the risk factors for coronary artery disease?

- Positive family history (onset before age 50)
- Dyslipidemia
- Tobacco abuse
- Hypertension
- Physical inactivity
- Obesity
- Diabetes mellitus
- Low estrogen levels in women
- Men over the age of 45
- Women over the age of 55

2. When should a patient be screened for cardiovascular disease?

The current recommendation is that a comprehensive risk assessment and complete lipoprotein profile be done at age 20 and every 5 years thereafter.

3. What is acute coronary syndrome (ACS)?

ACS is a term that is broadly used to describe a variety of coronary disorders such as unstable angina, non-ST-elevation myocardial infarction, and ST-elevation myocardial infarction.

4. What is the difference between stable and unstable angina?

Angina symptoms are defined as stable when there is no substantial change or worsening of symptoms over several weeks. For example, a man only has symptoms when he plays racquetball, but can perform all other activities.

Unstable angina is any new-onset angina or when the symptom pattern changes abruptly. For example, the same gentleman above suddenly develops chest pain when carrying the trash bag to the end of the driveway, and the next morning has pain while showering.

5. **What is the incidence and prevalence of acute coronary syndrome?**

ACS accounts for 2 million hospitalizations and 30% of deaths each year in the United States.

6. **What is the incidence and prevalence of myocardial infarction (MI)?**

Each year about 1.1 million Americans suffer a heart attack. About 460,000 of those heart attacks are fatal. About half of those deaths occur within 1 hour of the start of symptoms and before the person reaches the hospital.

Every 28.7 seconds, 1 American has an MI. In an 8-hour workday, 1003 Americans will have an MI.

7. **What are the present ACC and AHA Class I recommendations for the evaluation of chest pain?**

Patients with suspected acute coronary syndrome (ACS) with chest discomfort at rest for greater than 20 minutes and/or patients with hemodynamic instability or recent syncope or presyncope should be strongly considered for immediate referral to any emergency room or to a specialized chest pain unit.
   - Assess likelihood of coronary artery disease
   - Assess risks of adverse events

8. **What are the classifications of angina?**

Angina is classified according to the Canadian classification system.
   - Class I: Ordinary physical activity does not cause angina. Symptoms only occur with extremes in physical exertion.
   - Class II: Patient reports a slight limitation in their everyday activities. Symptoms occur from walking more than 2 blocks on a level surface or climbing more than 1 flight of stairs at a normal pace.
   - Class III: Patient reports a marked limitation in their ordinary physical activity. Symptoms occur from walking 1 to 2 blocks on a flat surface or climbing 1 flight of stairs at a normal pace.
   - Class IV: Patient reports an inability to perform any activity without discomfort. Symptoms occur at rest or with minimal exertion.

9. **What are the classic symptoms associated with angina?**
   - Chest pain
   - Substernal pain, possibly radiating to the neck or back
   - Back pain
   - Jaw pain
   - Arm heaviness and/or numbness
   - Pain that can be described as squeezing, crushing, heavy, or aching
   - Pain lasting at least 15 minutes
   - Pain may be of moderate or severe intensity
   - Shortness of breath

- Syncope
- Dyspnea

10. What are the atypical symptoms of angina?

- Fatigue
- Weakness
- Flulike symptoms
- Malaise
- Heart failure
- Hypertension and/or hypertensive crisis
- Nausea/vomiting
- Low-grade fever
- Insomnia
- Indigestion
- Diaphoresis
- Orthopnea
- Paroxysmal nocturnal dyspnea
- Toothache (dentist cannot determine the cause)

11. What are some of the differential diagnoses for chest pain?

Anterior chest wall syndrome: inflammation of the chondrocostal junctions; pain described as sharp and localized

Tietze's syndrome: diffuse chest pain reproduced by local pressure

Cervical or thoracic spine disease: involves dorsal roots; related to specific movements of the neck or spine; pain occurs while lying, straining, or lifting

Peptic ulcer disease (PUD), cholecystitis, esophageal spasm, gastroesophageal reflux disease (GERD): typically relieved by antacids, carafate, H_2-receptor antagonists, or proton pump inhibitors; characterized by upper abdominal/lower chest discomfort after heavy meals or recumbent positioning. If gastric motility problems are present, it is difficult to differentiate because pain can be relieved with nitrates and calcium channel blockers.

Thoracic outlet syndrome: irritation of nerves or muscular compression; symptoms precipitated by movement of the arm and/or shoulder; often associated with paresthesias

Spontaneous pneumothorax: most often seen in young, tall African-American males; characterized by chest pain and shortness of breath; ECG changes may be seen

Pneumonia: pain typically with deep inspiration

Pulmonary embolism: pain typically with deep inspiration

Pleurisy: usually unilateral pain described as knifelike and superficial; pain aggravated by cough or deep inspiration

Pericarditis: steady crushing, substernal pain; often has a pleuritic component characterized by pain with cough or deep inspiration

Aortic dissection: extreme and severe midsternal chest or back pain, described as "ripping feeling" in chest; may be associated with loss of peripheral pulses or substantial difference between arm and leg blood pressures

Disorder	Characterization of Pain
Anterior chest wall syndrome	Sharp and localized
Tietze's syndrome	Diffuse chest pain reproduced by local pressure
Cervical or thoracic spine disease	Pain related to movement of neck or spine
Peptic ulcer disease, esophageal spasms, gastroesophageal reflux disease, and cholecystitis	Pain typically relieved by antacids; upper abdominal pain and lower chest pain after eating or lying in recumbent position
Thoracic outlet syndrome	Pain associated with movement of arm and shoulder, associated with paresthesia
Spontaneous pneumothorax	Chest pain and shortness of breath
Pneumonia	Pain typically with deep inspiration
Pulmonary embolism	Pain typically with deep inspiration
Pleurisy	Unilateral, knifelike pain, worsened by cough or deep inspiration
Pericarditis	Steady crushing, substernal pain
Aortic dissection	Severe midsternal chest or back pain

12. **What are the physical exam findings that may be found in an individual experiencing an acute myocardial infarction?**
    - Distant S_1 and S_2
    - New S_4
    - S_3 with left ventricular failure
    - Crackles
    - Clenching fist over chest
    - Facial grimacing
    - Apprehension
    - Diaphoresis
    - Pallor

13. **How is the diagnosis of myocardial infarction made?**

    The 12-lead electrocardiogram (ECG) is the gold standard in the diagnosis of acute myocardial infarction (AMI). The ECG may reveal:
    - ST-segment elevation or a new left bundle branch block (LBBB) has a high specificity for evaluating infarcted tissue.
    - ST-segment depression is strongly suggestive of ischemic coronary tissue; it defines a high-risk group of patients with non-Q-wave myocardial infarctions (NQWMIs) or unstable angina.
    - With a nondiagnostic or normal ECG, continue monitoring ECG and perform serial cardiac injury panel markers; an echocardiogram or exercise stress test may be needed.
    - Echocardiogram: Regional wall motion abnormalities are seen in the presence of infarcted myocardial tissue.

- Cardiac markers become elevated in the presence of cellular death.
- Achieve early diagnosis; early peak in levels provides prognostic indication that complications will occur and will also differentiate between NQWMI and unstable angina. CK-MB isoenzymes are early markers for myocardial necrosis.
- Cardiac troponins: troponin-I and troponin-T are proteins not normally detected and are present with minimal damage in patients with unstable angina. These patients are at high risk for subsequent nonfatal MI or sudden cardiac death.
- C-Reactive protein: There is evolving evidence that shows inflammatory markers can indicate plaque or systemic inflammation associated with acute coronary syndromes. A positive C-reactive protein in individuals with unstable angina shows those individuals to be at high risk for adverse cardiac events.

14. **What is the initial management of myocardial infarction?**
- Cardiac catheterization and revascularization in moderate- to high-risk patients
- Fibrinolytic therapy (when cardiac catherization lab and angioplasty not available)
- Vasodilator administration: nitrates and morphine
- Heparin or low molecular weight heparin administration
- Oxygen use
- Aspirin administration: chewable
- Beta-blocker administration: use cautiously in the acute phase
- ACE inhibitor administration: typically begun within 6 to 24 hours after infarction stabilized
- Assess lipid panel and implement therapy

15. **What are the current recommendations with regard to the use of thrombolytic therapy in the treatment of myocardial infarctions?**
- Chest pain suggesting an acute myocardial infarction
- ST-segment elevation >0.1 mV (1 mm) in two or more contiguous leads, or new or presumably new LBBB, strongly suggestive of injury (bundle branch block [BBB] obscures ST-segment analysis)
- Chest pain of less than 12-hours duration
- Age <75 years

16. **What are the contraindications for thrombolytic therapy?**
Absolute:
- Previous hemorrhagic stroke
- Stroke or transient ischemic attack within last year
- Active internal bleeding (menses excluded)
- Suspected aortic dissection

Relative:
- Uncontrolled HTN (>180/110 mm Hg)
- Current use of anticoagulation therapy (INR >2.5)
- Known bleeding disorder
- Recent trauma within 2 to 4 weeks (included cardiopulmonary resuscitation [CPR])

- Major surgery within last 3 weeks
- Internal bleeding within last 4 weeks
- Active peptic ulcer disease (PUD)
- Pregnancy

17. **What antiplatelet agents are available in the management of acute coronary syndrome (ACS)?**

    Aspirin: Thromboxane A_2 receptor antagonist; selectively inhibits the binding of thromboxane A_2 to its platelet receptor

    Clopidogrel (Plavix): Adenosine diphosphate (ADP) receptor antagonist; selectively inhibits the binding of ADP to its platelet receptor

    Ticlopidine (Ticlid): ADP receptor antagonist; inhibits ADP-induced platelet fibrinogen binding

    Glycoprotein IIb/IIIa (GPIIb/IIIa) inhibitors

    Abciximab (ReoPro): A monoclonal antibody derived from mice antibodies; it is FDA-approved for the management of non-Q-wave myocardial infarctions (NQWMI), acute coronary syndromes (ACS), and unstable angina where percutaneous intervention is planned within 24 hours of presentation

    Eptifibatide (Integrilin): A cyclic heptapeptide that binds to the receptor; it is FDA-approved for the management of NQWMI or unstable angina that is being managed medically

    Tirofiban (Aggrastat): A synthetic nonpeptide; it is FDA-approved for the management of ACS

    Lotrafiban, Orofiban, and Sirofiban: Oral GPIIb/IIIa inhibitors that were in clinical trials; these trials were abruptly stopped because of the increased number of cardiac events suffered by those individuals given the medication

18. **Is there evidence to suggest that clopidogrel (Plavix) can reduce the incidence of cardiac events?**

    In CURE, a clinical trial, dual antiplatelet therapy of aspirin and Plavix resulted in a 20% to 30% reduction in cardiovascular death, myocardial infarction, and stroke when compared to aspirin alone in those patients with non-ST-elevation acute coronary syndromes.

19. **What role do glycoprotein IIb/IIIa inhibitors have in the management of ACS?**

    - Inhibit the Integrilin GPIIb/IIIa receptors in the membrane of platelets
    - Inhibit the common final pathway in the activation of platelet aggregation

20. **What are the contraindications for the use of GPIIb/IIIa inhibitors?**

    - Active internal bleeding
    - Recent gastrointestinal or genitourinary bleeding (within last 6 weeks) that has been clinically significant

- History of cerebrovascular accident (CVA) within the last 2 years, or any CVA that has left a significant neurovascular deficit
- History of intracranial hemorrhage, intracranial neoplasm, arteriovenous malformation, or aneurysm
- Bleeding diathesis
- History of thrombocytopenia following prior exposure to any of the GPIIb/IIIa inhibitors
- Any major surgical procedure or severe physical trauma within the previous 6 weeks
- History, symptoms, or findings suggestive of aortic dissection
- Severe hypertension (systolic blood pressure >180 mm Hg and/or diastolic blood pressure >110 mm Hg)
- Acute pericarditis
- Known hypersensitivity to any component of the product (for example, ReoPro is contraindicated in those individuals sensitive or allergic to murine products)
- Thrombocytopenia (<100,000 cells per microliter)
- Presumed or documented history of vasculitis
- Relative contraindication: Administration of oral anticoagulants within 7 days before administration of GPIIb/IIIa inhibitors unless the prothrombin time is less than 1.5 times the control (INR <1.5)
- Relative contraindication: Use of intravenous dextran before administration of GPIIb/IIIa inhibitors

21. How do you differentiate an ST-elevation from a non-ST-elevation myocardial infarction?

Electrocardiogram Changes in AMI

• ST elevation >1 mm in at least two consecutive leads	• ST depression >0.5 mm and/or T-wave inversion >2 mm indicate high risk • Nonspecific ST changes or a normal ECG may be seen
• Q waves develop in approximately 80% of these patients	• Q waves develop in approximately 20% of these patients

22. How reliable is the 12-lead electrocardiogram in the diagnosis of myocardial infarctions?

The initial ECG is diagnostic of acute infarction in approximately 50% of the population. In 40% of the population it is abnormal, but not diagnostic for infarction patterns. It may be normal in 10% of patients that have symptoms of an acute MI.

23. What are the vectorcardiographic criteria for the diagnosis of myocardial infarction?

Type AMI	Affected Artery	Region	ECG Finding
Anterior	LAD or branches	Anterior wall of LV, LBB, RBB, 23 septum, bundle of His	V_3-V_4: Q waves V_2-V_6: R-wave progression not present
Anteroseptal	LAD	Anterior wall of LV, intraventricular	V_1-V_4: Q waves Poor R-wave progression
Inferior	RCA or dominant circumflex artery	Inferior or diaphragmatic LV wall	II, III, aV_F: new or deepened Q waves, ST elevation, or inverted T waves
Posterior infarct	RCA Circumflex	Posterior left ventricle	V_1-V_2: reciprocal changes, ST segment depression; R waves tall, reversed polls
RV infarct	Distal RCA	Right ventricle, left ventricle inferior wall	II, III, aV_F, V_{3E}, V_{4R}: ST elevation and Q waves
Lateral wall infarct	Circumflex LAD	Lateral wall, left ventricle	I, aV_L, V_5, V_6: new or deeper Q waves, ST segment elevation

24. What is the role of myocardial perfusion imaging or stress imaging (nuclide/echocardiogram) in patients presenting with angina?

The basic principle of stress imaging is to provoke ischemia of myocardial tissue followed by functional assessment of the heart using a variety of different testing strategies. Exercise is the most effective way to induce ischemia and also assists in grading angina according to the Canadian classification system. Pharmacologic testing can be used in those patients who cannot effectively exercise.

25. What are the indications for coronary catheterization?

- Acute coronary infarction
- Recurrent ischemia
- Left ventricular (LV) dysfunction (ejection fraction $\leq 40\%$)
- Unstable angina
- Congestive heart failure
- Hemodynamic instability

- Valvular disease (especially if new murmur)
- Prior MI or CABG
- Inability to exercise
- Ventricular tachycardia (VT) >48 hours after MI
- Ischemia, arrhythmia, or hypotension during an exercise stress test
- Thoracic aneurysm
- Inadequate control of symptoms despite optimal medical therapy
- Suspected coronary artery dissection

26. What are the benefits of percutaneous transluminal coronary angioplasty (PTCA)?

- Reduced number of myocardial infarctions
- Reduced incidence of intracranial hemorrhage
- Reduced number of deaths postinfarction
- Reduced rates of reinfarction
- Reduced incidence of CVAs (benefits occur early and are sustained up to 6 months)

27. What are some of the complications of PTCA?

- Reperfusion dysrhythmias
- Bleeding
- Ischemia (coronary or limb)
- Infection
- Adverse reactions to intravenous contrast or medications
- Myocardial infarction
- Cerebral vascular accident
- Death

28. When should pacing be considered in a patient having an acute myocardial infarction?

Prophylactic pacing is recommended to prevent hemodynamic collapse in the event that the conduction delay progresses to tertiary atrioventricular block (AVB).

29. What dysrhythmias could be seen with an acute myocardial infarction?

- Mobitz II secondary AVB
- New left or right bundle branch block (LBBB/RBBB)
- Left anterior or posterior fascicular block (LAFB/LPFB)
- Ventricular tachycardia (VT)
- Ventricular fibrillation (VF)

30. What are the indications for intraaortic balloon pumping?

- Cardiogenic shock
- Refractory chest pain not responding to traditional medical therapy

- Stabilizing bridge to surgical repair of a ruptured papillary muscle, ventricular-septal defect, or chordae tendineae
- Significant left main trunk disease
- Severe triple-vessel disease with poor LV function
- Hypotension (peri-infarct)

31. What are the contraindications for intraaortic balloon pumping?

- Aortic insufficiency (moderate to severe)
- Aortic dissection
- Severe peripheral vascular disease
- Descending aortic or peripheral vascular grafts
- Abdominal or thoracic aneurysm

32. What is cardiogenic shock?

It is a state that occurs when the heart is no longer able to effectively pump blood, resulting in inadequate tissue perfusion. This occurs when there is oxygen deprivation to the myocardium and consequent tissue damage to the right and/or left ventricle of the heart.

33. What are the causes of cardiogenic shock?

- Primary ventricular ischemia
- Acute myocardial infarction
- Cardiopulmonary arrest
- Open heart surgery
- Structural abnormalities
  - Septal, papillary, or free wall rupture
  - Ventricular aneurysms or tumors
  - Cardiomyopathies
  - Pulmonary embolism
  - Valvular dysfunction
  - Cardiac tamponade (with or without free wall rupture)
  - Myocardial contusion
- Dysrhythmias (tachy or brady)
- Aortic dissection
- Myocarditis

34. What is the management approach in cardiogenic shock?

- Treat the underlying cause
- Enhance the effectiveness of the pump
- Improve tissue perfusion

35. What noninvasive testing may be ordered to assess the severity of coronary artery disease in a patient with anginal complaints?

- Exercise stress test
- Pharmacological stress test (Persantine, adenosine, dobutamine)
- Echocardiogram
- CAT scan with calcium score

36. When is coronary artery bypass grafting (CABG) considered in the presence of an acute myocardial infarction?

- Left main stenosis >50% with left anterior descending or left circumflex coronary infarct vessel
- Left main stenosis >75% with right coronary infarct vessel
- Severe proximal multivessel disease not amenable to percutaneous angioplasty
- Severe multivessel disease with cardiogenic shock
- Ongoing ischemic pain despite intraaortic balloon pump and maximized medical therapy

37. What is a right ventricular (RV) infarct?

An RV infarct occurs as a result of an occlusion of the right coronary artery. It is seen in 30% to 50% of patients who suffer an inferior-posterior MI. The incidence of an isolated RV infarct is rare, although possible; 10% of patients with an RV infarct show hemodynamic compromise.

38. What pharmacological agents should be part of the discharge medication regime for a patient who has recently suffered an MI?

- Aspirin
- Plavix
- Beta-blocker
- ACE inhibitor
- Statin

39. What risk factor modifications should be made in individuals with coronary artery disease?

- Age, sex, and family history cannot be modified
- Reduction of excess weight
- Eat a healthy diet
- Start an exercise program
- Aggressive lipid management using present guidelines
- Smoking cessation
- Stress management
- Diabetes management

Key Points

- Acute coronary syndrome represents a variety of coronary disorders such as unstable angina, non-ST-elevation myocardial infarction, and ST-elevation myocardial infarction.
- Risk factors associated with coronary artery disease include family history, dyslipidemia, hypertension, obesity, diabetes mellitus, smoking, men greater than 45 years of age, women greater than 55 years of age.

The classification of angina is the Canadian classification system:

- Class I: Ordinary physical activity does not cause angina. Symptoms only occur with extremes in physical exertion.

- Class II: Patient reports a slight limitation in their everyday activities. Symptoms occur from walking more than 2 blocks on a level surface or climbing more than 1 flight of stairs at a normal pace.

- Class III: Patient reports a marked limitation in their ordinary physical activity. Symptoms occur from walking 1 to 2 blocks on a flat surface or climbing 1 flight of stairs at a normal pace.

- Class IV: Patient reports an inability to perform any activity without discomfort. Symptoms occur at rest or with minimal exertion.

Internet Resources

Guidant: For Patients and Families: Coronary Artery Disease—At A Glance:
http://www.guidant.com/condition/cad/condition.html

Cardiothoracic Surgery Notes: Coronary Artery Disease:
http://www.ctsnet.org/residents/ctsn/archives/not32.html

Bibliography

2002 ACC/AHA UA/NSTEMI Guideline Update: available at www.acc.org, 2002.

Braunwald E: *Heart Disease: A Textbook of Cardiovascular Medicine*, ed 5, Philadelphia, 1997, WB Saunders.

Califf RM: *ACS Essentials*, Mich, 2003, Physician Press.

Cor Therapeutics and Key Pharmaceuticals: www.integrilin.com, 2000.

Eli-Lilly: www.reopro.com, 2000.

Gawlinski A, Hamwi D: *Acute Care Nurse Practitioner: Clinical Curriculum and Certification Review*, Philadelphia, 1999, WB Saunders.

Grimes C: Presentation at ACC, Beamont University Hospital, March 2003.

Hazinski MF, Cummins RO, Field JM: *Handbook of Emergency Cardiovascular Care*, American Heart Association, Tex, 2000.

Isselbacher KJ, Braunwald E, Wilson JD, Martin JB, Fauci AS, Kasper DL: *Harrison's Principles of Internal Medicine*, ed 13, New York, 1995, McGraw-Hill.

Marso SP, Griffin BP, Topol EJ: *Manual of Cardiovascular Medicine*, Philadelphia, 2000, Lippincott Williams & Wilkins.

Merck: www.aggrastat.com, 2003.

Parillo JE, Bone RC: *Critical Care Medicine: Principles of Diagnosis and Management*, Philadelphia, 1995, Mosby.

Transcatheter Cardiovascular Institute (TCT): CD Rom Collection, Lenox Hill Heart and Vascular Institute of New York, 2002.

Valvular Heart Disease

Barbara A. Todd and V. Paul Addonizio

1. **How many valves are found in the heart?**

   The heart has four valves. There are two valves for the left heart and two valves for the right heart.

2. **Name the atrioventricular (AV) valves.**
   - Tricuspid valve
   - Mitral valve

3. **Name the semilunar valves.**
   - Aortic valve
   - Pulmonic valve

4. **How many leaflets are present in each valve?**

   Every valve inside the heart contains three leaflets. The only exception is the mitral valve, which contains two leaflets. Congenital anomalies, however, produce many variants of this main theme. Valves that are normally trileaflet, but at birth are bileaflet, are probably the most common congenital abnormality. However, valves can contain extra leaflets. Valves with fewer or extra leaflets rarely function normally.

5. **Describe the functional abnormalities that can affect the cardiac valves.**

   The cardiac valves are susceptible to only two types of functional abnormalities. Valves may gradually provide an ever-increasing obstruction to the flow of blood across them. This condition is called valvular stenosis. Valves may also become incompetent, no longer preventing the reversal of the flow of blood. This condition is called valvular regurgitation. A given abnormal valve can have elements of both stenosis and regurgitation.

6. **What causes valvular incompetence?**

   - Congenital abnormalities
   - Myxomatous degeneration
   - Infections (endocarditis)
   - Pharmacological agents (for example, Phen-Phen)
   - Radiation exposure
   - Cardiac failure with ventricular chamber dilatation

7. **What is valvular regurgitation?**

   Valvular regurgitation is incomplete closure of the cardiac valves, thus allowing backflow of blood.

8. **What are the hemodynamic sequelae of abnormally functioning valves?**

Valvular Lesion	Hemodynamic Sequelae
Aortic regurgitation	Left ventricular dilatation
Aortic stenosis	Left ventricular hypertrophy
Pulmonic regurgitation	Right ventricular dilatation
Pulmonic stenosis	Right ventricular hypertrophy
Mitral regurgitation	Left ventricular dilatation
Mitral stenosis	Left atrial dilatation
Tricuspid regurgitation	Right atrial and ventricular dilatation
Tricuspid stenosis	Right ventricular hypertrophy

9. **What causes valvular stenosis?**

   - Congenital abnormalities (too few cusps)
   - Acquired pathologies (calcification, rheumatic fever)

10. **What are valvular gradients?**

    The additional pressure required to drive blood across a valve, which provides an obstruction, is called the pressure gradient. For example, if a systemic pressure in the aorta of 120 mm Hg is considered normal and the aortic valve provides an obstruction, the pressure over and above the systemic pressure that the ventricular chamber must generate to drive the blood would be called the gradient. A simple example makes this easier to understand. If the systemic aortic pressure is 120 mm Hg during systole and at the same moment, with the valve open, the pressure in the left ventricular chamber is 200 mm Hg, then the gradient would be 80 mm Hg. This means that the ventricle must generate 80 mm Hg additional pressure to drive the blood across the valve to obtain the 120 mm Hg pressure, which would be considered normal in the aorta. Up to a point, as the valvular diameter decreases the gradient increases. Eventually, however, the ventricles become exhausted and compensate, not by increasing muscle mass and generating increasing pressure, but by dilating. When this occurs the ventricles begin to fail and gradients actually decrease. This is not a measure of improvement, but an ominous sign indicating that compensatory mechanisms have failed.

11. **How are cardiac valve problems diagnosed?**

Cardiac valve problems are diagnosed by a multifaceted analysis, as are most other clinical situations:
- Physical examination
- Cardiac auscultation
- Clinical history
- Chest x-ray
- Echocardiogram:
  - Transthoracic
  - Transesophageal
- Hemodynamic monitoring
- Cardiac catherization

12. **What are treatment options for cardiac valve problems?**

- Medical management; administration of:
  - Nitrates
  - Beta-blockers
  - ACE inbibitors
  - ACE receptor blockers
  - Anticoagulants
  - Lanoxin
  - Inotropes
- Intraaortic balloon pumping
- Valvuloplasty (for stenotic valves)
- Surgical management:
  - Valvular reconstruction
  - Valve replacement

13. **During which phase of the cardiac cycle do the heart valves open?**

The tricuspid and mitral valves open during the diastolic phase, which is the period of ventricular filling. The pulmonic and aortic valves open during systole, which is the period of ejection of blood from the heart.

14. **What are common symptoms associated with valvular heart disease?**

- Exertional fatigue
- Tachycardia

- Syncope
- Presyncopal episodes
- Chest pain
- Dyspnea

15. **What is aortic regurgitation?**

Aortic regurgitation is a valvular disorder in which the aortic valve allows blood to flow back into the left ventricle from the aorta.

16. **What are common mechanisms associated with chronic aortic regurgitation?**

- Hypertension
- Rheumatic heart disease
- Endocarditis
- Congenital bicuspid valve abnormalities
- Autoimmune disorders
- Marfan syndrome

17. **What are common findings in patients with aortic regurgitation?**

- Widened pulse pressure
- Low diastolic blood pressure
- Palpitations
- Flushing
- Shortness of breath
- Ventricular gallop
- Diastolic murmur heard at the left sternal border
- Crackles

18. **What is the most common congenital cardiac valve problem?**

Bicuspid aortic valve stenosis

19. **What is the triad of symptoms commonly associated with aortic stenosis?**

- Syncope
- Angina
- Dyspnea

20. **What are the physical exam findings associated with aortic stenosis?**

- Crescendo-decrescendo systolic murmur
- Laterally displaced apical impulse

- Possible atrial gallop (S_4)
- Decreased carotid upstroke

21. What are the common causes of aortic stenosis?

- Congenital abnormal valve
- Calcification
- Rheumatic fever

22. What considerations should be given to patients who have aortic stenosis?

Use of pharmacological agents that will decrease preload, such as diuretics and vasodilators, should be carefully monitored.

23. What is the most common cause of mitral stenosis?

Rheumatic fever

24. What are common symptoms associated with mitral stenosis?

- Fatigue
- Decreased exercise tolerance
- Shortness of breath
- Hemoptysis
- Paroxysmal nocturnal dyspnea (PND)

25. What are the auscultatory findings in mitral stenosis?

- Opening snap in early diastole
- Rumbling diastolic murmur at the apex
- Loud first heart sound

26. What is rheumatic fever?

Rheumatic fever is an acute inflammatory disease that is a complication of group A streptococcal upper respiratory infection.

27. What are the cardiac manifestations of rheumatic fever?

- Myocarditis
- Endocarditis
- Pericarditis

28. Which cardiac valves are most often affected by rheumatic fever?

- Mitral valve
- Aortic valve

29. What are the major and minor diagnostic criteria for rheumatic fever?

Major Criteria	Minor Criteria
Carditis	Fever
Polyarthritis	Migratory arthralgias
Chorea	Elevated C-reactive protein
Subcutaneous nodules	Elevated erythrocyte sedimentation rate
Erythema marginatum	Heart block

30. What are the recommendations for secondary prevention of rheumatic fever?

Penicillin G should be given, 1.2 million units intramuscularly every 4 weeks, OR penicillin, 250 mg orally twice daily. If the patient is allergic to penicillin, then give erythromycin, 250 mg orally twice daily.

The duration of therapy is dependent on the extent of cardiac involvement; it may range from 5 to 10 years to lifelong therapy.

31. What are some of the most common causes of mitral regurgitation?

- Myxomatous degeneration of the mitral valve
- Rheumatic fever
- Coronary artery disease
- Bacterial endocarditis
- Mitral valve prolapse

32. What are the hemodynamic effects associated with mitral regurgitation?

- Acute volume overload
- Increased left ventricle (LV) preload
- Increased LV stroke volume
- Decreased forward stroke volume
- Decreased cardiac output
- Pulmonary edema

33. Describe the cardiac sound associated with mitral regurgitation.

A holosystolic murmur may be heard at the apex of the heart and it may radiate to the axilla and the posterior chest wall.

34. What treatment regimens may be instituted in patients with mitral regurgitation?

- Use of diuretics
- Vasodilator therapies: angiotensin-converting enzyme inhibitors and blockers

- Use of anticoagulants
- Intraaortic balloon pump therapy
- Surgical interventions including mitral valve reconstruction or replacement

35. **What is the most common dysrhythmia associated with mitral valve disease?**

Atrial fibrillation

36. **What is mitral valve prolapse (MVP) syndrome?**

This syndrome is a genetic connective tissue disorder that primarily affects the mitral valve leaflets, chordae, and annulus. There are thickened leaflets with systolic displacement into the left atrium.

37. **What are some of the sequelae of mitral valve prolapse (MVP) syndrome?**

- Atypical chest pain
- Embolic events
- Infective endocarditis
- Progressive mitral regurgitation
- Sudden cardiac death secondary to arrhythmias

38. **What are the classic cardiac auscultatory findings associated with MVP?**

- Midsystolic click
- Late systolic murmur

39. **Describe the management of MVP.**

For most patients, no treatment is warranted. However, if they are symptomatic with chest pain and palpations, beta-blockers may be instituted.

If there is mitral regurgitation, then endocarditis prophylaxis is recommended.

40. **What are some of the primary causes of tricuspid regurgitation?**

- Rheumatic fever
- Myxomatous degeneration
- Endocarditis
- Carcinoid tumor
- Ebstein's anomaly
- Trauma
- Endomyocardial fibrosis
- Iatrogenesis

41. **What are some of the secondary causes of tricuspid regurgitation?**
    - Primary pulmonary hypertension
    - Chronic pulmonary disease
    - Left ventricular heart disease

42. **What are the physical examination findings associated with tricuspid regurgitation?**
    - Jugular vein distention
    - Peripheral edema
    - Hepatomegaly
    - Holosystolic murmur heard at the left sternal border, and increased with inspiration

43. **What is the most common surgical treatment for tricuspid regurgitation?**
    Tricuspid valve annuloplasty

44. **What is the cardiac valve most often affected with endocarditis in patients with intravenous drug use?**
    Tricuspid valve

45. **What is the most common cause of tricuspid stenosis?**
    Rheumatic fever

46. **What is the most common cause of pulmonic stenosis (PS)?**
    Congenital abnormality

47. **What are the common symptoms associated with PS?**
    - Fatigue
    - Dyspnea

48. **Describe the cardiac murmur associated with PS.**
    The murmur is a crescendo-decrescendo systolic murmur auscultated loudest at the upper left sternal border and radiating to the suprasternal notch and neck.

49. **What is the most common cause of pulmonary regurgitation in the adult?**
    - Pulmonary artery dilatation secondary to pulmonary hypertension
    - Pulmonic valve annular dilatation

50. **Describe the cardiac murmur associated with pulmonic regurgitation.**

This murmur is usually a soft, diastolic murmur heard best at the left upper parasternal region.

51. **What is infective endocarditis?**

Infective endocarditis is an inflammation of the endocardium caused by invasion of microorganisms.

52. **What are the cardiac abnormalities that may predispose to the development of endocarditis?**
    - Native valve disease
    - Congenital heart defects
    - Ventricular and atrial septal defects
    - Coarctation of the aorta
    - Patent ductus arteriosus
    - Eisenmenger's syndrome
    - Cardiomyopathy
    - Prosthetic heart valves

53. **What are the classic peripheral manifestations associated with endocarditis?**
    - Osler's nodes (tiny bluish nodules on the fingertips, usually painful)
    - Janeway's lesions (small pink macules on the fingertips, painless)
    - Roth's spots (areas of retinal bleeding)

54. **What are the treatment options for native valve endocarditis?**
    - Medical management (antibiotics and heart failure management)
    - Surgical management

55. **What are the indications for surgery in native valve endocarditis?**
    - Persistent bacteremia
    - Embolization
    - Valvular destruction
    - Heart failure

56. Describe the physical examination findings in patients with valvular heart disease.

Lesion	Murmur	S_1	S_2	Associated Findings	Maneuver
Aortic stenosis	Midsystolic to late systolic, may be soft or absent if severe	Normal	Single or paradoxically split	Diminished carotid upstroke, S_3, S_4	Softer with Valsalva maneuver
Aortic regurgitation	Blowing diastolic	Soft	Normal	Wide pulse pressure, systolic HTN, brisk carotid upstroke	Murmur increased with handgrip or squatting
Mitral regurgitation	Holosystolic	Soft	Normal or split	S_3, crackles, hyperdynamic PMI	Louder with Valsalva maneuver
Mitral stenosis	Diastolic rumble	Loud	Normal	Opening snap	Increased during exercise
Mitral valve prolapse	Midsystolic to late systolic	Normal	Normal	Midsystolic click	Increased with standing
Tricuspid regurgitation	Holosystolic	Loud	Normal or split	Right ventricular S_3, hepatomegaly, edema, JVD	Increased with inspiration
Tricuspid stenosis	Diastolic rumbling murmur heard at right sternal border	Loud	Absent or widely split	Opening snap	Murmur be may inaudible
Pulmonic regurgitation	Soft diastolic, decrescendo murmur	Normal	Widely split	Right ventricular heave	None
Pulmonic stenosis	Crescendo-decrescendo systolic murmur loudest at left upper sternal border	Normal	Widely split S_2	Ejection click, palpable thrill, right ventricular hypertrophy	None

Key Points

- Common symptoms associated with aortic stenosis are syncope, angina and dyspnea.
- The most common cause of mitral stenosis is rheumatic fever.
- Valvular regurgitation can be caused by congenital abnormalities, chamber dilatation, infection, and myxomatous degeneration.

 Internet Resources

ACC/AHA Guidelines for the Management of Patients with Valvular Heart Disease:
http://www.acc.org/clinical/guidelines/valvular

Heart Center Online: For Cardiologists and Their Patients:
http://www.heartcenteronline.com

Bibliography

Bonow R, Carabello B, et al: ACC/AHA Guidelines for the Management of Patients with Valvular Disease, *JACC* 32(5):1446-1588, 1998.

Goldman L, Braunwald E: *Primary Cardiology*, Philadelphia, 1998, WB Saunders.

Griffin B, Hayek E: Current Medical Management of Valvular Heart Disease, *Clev Clin J Med* 10:881-887, 2001.

Otto C: *Valvular Heart Disease*, Philadelphia, 1999, WB Saunders.

Chapter 7

Aortic Dissection

Kathleen Shaughnessy

1. **What is the difference between an aneurysm and a dissection?**

   A dissection is a circumferential or transverse tear between the intima and media, causing a false channel in which blood can collect. An aneurysm is a pathological dilatation of the blood vessel layers (intima, media, and adventitia). Aneurysmal formation does not imply an early stage of dissection.

2. **How are thoracic dissections classified?**

   Dissections are classified according to location, originating in the ascending aorta, aortic arch, or descending aorta. The locations are further defined using two separate nomenclature classification systems. The Standford system includes type A and type B dissections. Type A involves the ascending aorta whether the tear has originated in the proximal aorta. A tear that originates in the descending aorta with retrograde arch extension is still considered a Type B dissection. Type B dissections involve the descending aorta (distal to the left subclavian artery) and do not extend proximally. A DeBakey type I tear occurs in the ascending aorta, just distal to the aortic valve. A DeBakey type II tear is limited to the ascending aorta. The origin of a DeBakey type III tear occurs beyond the aortic arch and may be further subdivided into type IIIa (dissection is limited to the thoracic aorta) and type IIIb (dissection extends below the diaphragm).

3. **What predisposing conditions are associated with the development of a dissection?**

   - Hypertension
   - Congenital anomalies such as coarctation of the aorta or congenital abnormal aortic valve
   - Iatrogenic trauma of the aorta such as that induced by cardiopulmonary bypass catheters, intraaortic balloon pumps, or catheter devices
   - Hormonal-mediated changes in the medial layer during third-trimester pregnancy
   - Collagen vascular disorders, such as Marfan syndrome

4. **Why is it important to rapidly diagnose a thoracic dissection?**

   Symptoms may be subtle or confused with other potential diagnoses. Mortality increases 1% per hour for each hour the diagnosis remains obscure.

5. **What diagnostic modalities are best used to confirm the presence of a dissection?**

Diagnostic modalities used to confirm the presence of dissection

Test	Advantage	Disadvantage
Transthoracic echocardiogram (TTE)	Able to visualize proximal aortic tears	Unable to visualize arch and descending aorta tears
Transesophageal echocardiogram (TEE)	Able to detect ascending and descending dissections	Invasive; less useful in assessing arch dissections
Magnetic resonance imaging (MRI)	Able to identify entry site and direction of blood flow in arch and descending dissections	Limited availability; longer imaging time; not suitable for unstable patient
CT scan	Able to detect anatomical location of tear	Contrast injection and potential for renal dysfunction
Aortogram	Able to detect presence of true or false lumen, extent of dissection	Potential contrast-mediated allergic reaction, worsening renal function

Data from Tierney LM, McPhee ST, Papadakis MA, editors: *2002 Current Medical Diagnosis and Treatment*, pp 488-490, Norwalk, Conn, 2002, Appleton and Lange.

---

6. **What are the common presenting symptoms of aortic dissection?**
   - The most commonly reported symptom is sudden onset of chest and back pain, which may follow a migratory pattern, indicating propagation of hematoma.
   - Syncope is an ominous sign reflecting aortic rupture or inominate branch artery occlusion.
   - Focal neurological signs reflect arterial occlusion of cerebral or spinal circulation.
   - Pulse deficit may indicate limb ischemia.
   - Acute aortic insufficiency (AI) is identified in 50% of proximal dissections. AI occurs because the hematoma alters the normal aortic contour, causing dilation of the aortic root and annulus. This dilation prevents normal coaptation of the aortic leaflets.

- Hypotension due to shock or tamponade occurs in 20% of patients with ascending aortic dissection.

7. **What are the clinical signs of aortic insufficiency?**

- Diastolic high pitched murmur
- Bounding pulses
- Widened pulse pressure
- Ventricular gallop
- Quincke's pulse (visible pulsations in the nail beds)
- Congestive heart failure

8. **What clinical significance does aortic insufficiency play in the setting of dissection?**

Aortic insufficiency indicates dilation of the aortic root and annulus and insufficient closure of the aortic leaflets. AI allows backward blood flow and pulmonary congestion, usually leading to congestive heart failure. AI indicates a need to progress quickly to surgery.

9. **What are the life-threatening complications of aortic dissection?**

- Myocardial infarction
- Cerebrovascular accident
- Renal failure
- Cardiac tamponade
- Aortic rupture
- Paralysis

10. **Why is it important to rule out a dissection process within the differential for chest pain?**

If a patient with an undiagnosed dissection is treated with thrombolytic agents, exsanguination will occur.

11. **What medical therapy is instituted for treatment of aortic dissection?**

Aggressive antihypertensive agents are used to maintain systolic blood pressure at 100 to 110 mm Hg. Vasodilators are used in conjunction with beta-blockers to reduce both the blood pressure and the propulsive force of ejected blood from the left ventricle. Lower blood pressure lessens the likelihood of further hematoma propagation.

12. **Why is pain control important within the setting of dissection?**

Pain will further elevate blood pressure and may indicate expanding dissection or compression of surrounding organs. Pain control will help to reduce blood pressure and place less stress against the arterial wall.

13. **What are the indications for surgical repair of a type B dissection?**
    - Intractable pain
    - Organ malperfusion due to branch artery occlusion
    - Growth rate

14. **What surgical technique is used to repair an ascending aortic dissection?**

    Ascending dissections are approached via a median sternotomy. Excising the entry site tear and replacing the proximal aorta with a Dacron tube graft surgically repairs proximal dissection without aortic valve involvement. The coronary arteries must also be dissected from the diseased native aorta and reimplanted into the Dacron graft.

15. **What surgical techniques can be used when the tear extends to the aortic valve?**

    Occasionally, using pledgeted mattress sutures to resuspend the commissures may restore aortic valve competence. This technique brings the wall between the true and false lumens back against the outer aortic wall. Often the aortic valve and the proximal aorta are replaced (the Bentall procedure). The aortic valve is replaced by either a mechanical or a bioprosthetic valve. Bioprosthetic options include allograft, porcine, or bovine valves.

16. **Why is deep hypothermic circulatory arrest employed when the aortic arch is dissected?**

    Circulatory arrest at 20° C reduces cerebral metabolism by 23%. This safety net allows time to replace the arch and reconnect the supraaortic vessels to the arch prosthesis.

17. **Why is there a risk of paraplegia when repairing a descending thoracic dissection?**

    The left subclavian artery gives rise to the vertebral artery from which the anterior spinal artery originates. If the aorta is clamped distal to the left subclavian artery, there may be decreased blood flow to the spinal arteries that supply the spinal column.

18. **What is the long-term prognosis for patients with a surgically treated dissection?**

    The 10-year survival rate is approximately 60%.

19. **Why do patients with surgical repair of dissection/aneurysm require long-term surveillance?**

Aortic dissection and aneurysmal formation are chronic disease entities requiring life-long observation. Surgical repair eliminates only a portion of the diseased vessel. Echocardiogram or CT scan is recommended at 6-month intervals to identify any further growth of the aorta.

Key Points

- Hypertension is the most common condition associated with aortic dissection.
- Common symptoms associated with aortic dissection are migratory chest and back pain, syncope, and focal neurological deficits.
- The most important aspect in the management of aortic dissection is control of blood pressure.

Internet Resources

Acute Aortic Dissection:
http://www.ctsnet.org/residents/ctsn/archives/not75.html

Nurse Week: Aortic Aneurysms—Time Bombs in the Body:
http://www.nurseweek.com/ce/ce42a.html

Bibliography

Braunwald E, Fauci AS, Kasper DL, editors: *Harrison's Principles of Internal Medicine*, ed 15, pp 1431-1433, New York, 2001, McGraw-Hill.

Braunwald E, Zipes D, Libby P, editors: *Heart Disease—Textbook of Cardiovascular Medicine*, ed 6, p 1431, Philadelphia, WB Saunders.

Edmonds LH, editor: *Cardiac Surgery in the Adult*, pp 1125-1155, New York, 1997, McGraw-Hill.

Fuster V, Alexander RW, O'Rourke RA, editors: *The Heart*, ed 10, pp 2384-2389, New York, 2001, McGraw-Hill.

Tierney LM, McPhee ST, Papadakis MA, editors: *2002 Current Medical Diagnosis and Treatment*, pp 488-490, Norwalk, Conn, 2002, Appleton and Lange.

Chapter 8

Cardiac Arrhythmias

Rose B. Shaffer and Annette Mitchell

1. **Why should patients be monitored in lead V_1 if possible?**

   The time from the beginning of ventricular activation to when the electrical impulse reaches an electrode is called the ventricular activation time. Because V_1 is over the right ventricle and V_6 is over the left ventricle, these two leads are helpful in determining ventricular activation times. V_1 and V_6 are unipolar leads. These leads are used to identify the morphology (shape) of the QRS complexes to help determine right bundle branch block (RBBB) from left bundle branch block (LBBB) and ventricular tachycardia (VT) from supraventricular tachycardia (SVT) with aberration.

2. **What are the modified chest leads (MCL) for monitoring?**

   The modified chest leads (MCL) are bipolar precordial leads that mimic the unipolar precordial leads. To make MCL1 using bipolar leads (mimicking V_1), the positive electrode is placed in the V_1 position on the chest, and the negative electrode is placed on the left shoulder, under the left clavicle. To make MCL6 (mimicking V_6), the negative electrode is placed on the left shoulder, under the clavicle, and the positive electrode is placed in the V_6 position. Since MCL1 and MCL6 mimic V_1 and V_6, respectively, they can also be used to distinguish between RBBB and LBBB and between VT and SVT with aberration. If given both options, the unipolar leads (V_1 and V_6) should be used.

3. **Which disease states predispose patients to develop atrial fibrillation?**

   - Valvular heart disease (especially mitral or tricuspid)
   - Coronary artery disease including myocardial infarction
   - Congestive heart failure
   - Dilated and hypertrophic cardiomyopathies
   - Hypertension
   - Postcardiac surgery
   - Inflammatory or infiltrative diseases such as amyloidosis or pericarditis
   - Congenital heart defects

- Alcoholism
- Carbon monoxide poisoning
- Postthoracic surgery
- Acute or chronic pulmonary disease
- Metabolic abnormalities (hypokalemia, hyperthyroidism, pheochromocytoma)
- Enhanced vagal tone

4. How is atrial fibrillation classified?

Atrial fibrillation is classified by its propensity for self-termination. Paroxysmal atrial fibrillation refers to recurrent atrial fibrillation that spontaneously terminates within 48 hours without intervention. Persistent atrial fibrillation requires chemical or electrical cardioversion to terminate the rhythm. Permanent atrial fibrillation (also referred to as chronic atrial fibrillation) does not terminate spontaneously and is refractory to attempts to cardiovert with medical therapy. In fact, medical therapy to control the rhythm should be abandoned.

5. What is meant by lone atrial fibrillation?

The term lone atrial fibrillation is used to describe atrial fibrillation when there is no associated underlying structural heart disease (verified by echocardiography) or a history of hypertension.

6. What is the treatment of lone atrial fibrillation?

In patients less than 60 years who have lone atrial fibrillation, aspirin is the treatment of choice because the risk of thromboembolism is very low.

7. Is it preferable to attempt to maintain rate control or rhythm control for long-term management of atrial fibrillation?

Atrial fibrillation can cause palpitations, decreased exercise tolerance, dyspnea, and fatigue. Additionally, patients in atrial fibrillation with concomitant heart disease are at high risk for thromboembolism and stroke. For years these have been convincing reasons to attempt to maintain sinus rhythm (rhythm control). Historically it was assumed that patients who remained in rate-controlled atrial fibrillation had poorer outcomes than those treated with medications to maintain sinus rhythm. However, in an attempt to maintain sinus rhythm, large doses of antiarrhythmic medications may be required until the patient converts to sinus rhythm or is unable to tolerate the side effects of the medications. If a patient fails antiarrhythmic therapy, then rate control becomes the approach to treatment.

To answer the question of whether rate control versus rhythm control is better for patients in persistent atrial fibrillation, two large randomized studies were completed. The North American study (Atrial Fibrillation Follow-up Investigation of Rhythm Management [AFFIRM]) and the European study in The Netherlands (Rate Control versus Electrical Cardioversion for Persistent

Arial Fibrillation) reported outcomes in over 4500 patients with persistent atrial fibrillation. They found that rhythm control provided no advantage over rate control with respect to survival. Based on these data, rate control or rhythm control may be used as the first-line treatment of persistent atrial fibrillation, but rhythm control can be abandoned early if results are not satisfactory. These studies demonstrated that it is not essential to prescribe a medication with a borderline risk/benefit ratio when the survival outcome is no different than the outcome observed when rhythm or rate control is used to treat atrial fibrillation.

8. **What is the rationale for using pulmonary vein ablation for treatment of atrial fibrillation?**

Almost all patients with paroxysmal or persistent atrial fibrillation have focal triggers, predominantly originating in the pulmonary veins, which can be isolated from the left atrium and ablated using a catheter approach with radiofrequency energy. More than 90% of pulmonary veins can be ablated along the ostial segments, guided by pulmonary vein potentials. When three to four pulmonary veins are isolated and ablated, a good clinical outcome (complete resolution or marked improvement in symptoms) can be achieved with a single procedure and without the need for antiarrhythmic therapy. In permanent (chronic) atrial fibrillation, the substrate that maintains atrial fibrillation is more dominant than that of the focal triggers in paroxysmal or persistent atrial fibrillation, making pulmonary vein ablation less likely to provide a good clinical outcome. Therefore treatment of patients with drug-refractory paroxysmal or persistent atrial fibrillation should not be delayed to the point where the atrial fibrillation becomes permanent.

9. **What is the MAZE procedure?**

It is a surgical procedure that consists of making incisions in the atrium in an effort to disrupt the reentrant circuits associated with atrial fibrillation. The goal is to restore the patient to normal sinus rhythm.

10. **Which patient subgroups are the best candidates for pulmonary vein ablation?**

Patients who qualify for pulmonary vein ablation are those restricted with multi-drug-resistant paroxysmal or persistent atrial fibrillation and less commonly those with multi-drug-resistant permanent (chronic) atrial fibrillation.

11. **What are the limitations of pulmonary vein ablation for the treatment of atrial fibrillation?**

- Lengthy procedure
- Potential for pulmonary vein thrombosis
- Potential for thromboembolism
- Recurrence of atrial fibrillation

12. What is sick sinus syndrome?

Sick sinus syndrome (SSS) includes problems with sinus impulse generation and conduction, failure of escape pacemakers lower in the conduction system, and a susceptibility to paroxysmal or chronic supraventricular tachycardias (SVTs). When bradycardia alternates with recurrent SVT or rapid atrial fibrillation, it is referred to as tachycardia-bradycardia syndrome.

13. What are the clinical features of sick sinus syndrome?

- Isolated sinus bradycardia in the absence of vagal stimulation
- Inappropriate sinus rates in response to exercise or stress
- Sudden prolonged sinus pauses, especially after premature atrial contractions or after an episode of atrial tachycardia
- Chronic atrial fibrillation with a rapid ventricular response followed by a slow ventricular response (unrelated to medications such as digitalis, beta-blockers, or calcium blockers)
- Paroxysms of atrial fibrillation or flutter alternating with bradycardia

14. What are the common symptoms associated with sick sinus syndrome (SSS)?

- Dizziness/light-headedness
- Fatigue
- Dyspnea on exertion
- Syncope or presyncope

15. What are the treatment options for SSS?

Symptomatic SSS involves using atropine until a transcutaneous or transvenous pacemaker is available if there are bradyarrhythmias. Definitive treatment involves placement of a permanent pacemaker. Tachyarrhythmias are treated with atrioventricular node blocking drugs.

16. What are the distinguishing characteristics of the different types of atrioventricular (AV) heart blocks?

AV block is divided into three categories: first-, second-, and third-degree heart block.

First-degree heart block involves prolongation of the PR interval, rather than an actual block in the conduction system. In first-degree AV block, the PR interval is prolonged to >0.20 seconds and does not change from beat to beat. Patients are hemodynamically stable, and no specific treatment is required.

Second-degree heart block involves some atrial impulses not being conducted to the ventricles. The QRS duration helps determine if the block is above or below the bundle of His. If the QRS duration is narrow, then the block is above the bundle of His, and if the QRS durations are prolonged, then the block is below the bundle of His. Second-degree AV block is divided into two types: Mobitz type I, also called AV Wenckebach, and Mobitz type II. In Mobitz type I, the PR interval progressively lengthens until one P wave is not conducted. After the nonconducted P wave, the cycle starts over again. This causes grouped beating with R-R interval shortening. The QRS duration is usually normal. This type of block is usually benign and does not progress to a more serious type of heart block. Observation is usually the treatment of choice. With Mobitz type II heart block, there are two or more sinus P waves for every QRS, which may be narrow or widened, depending on the level of the block. With Mobitz type II heart block, there are dropped QRS complexes, but ALL of the PR intervals of the conducted beats are the same and are NOT prolonged. Patients with this type of block are usually symptomatic, depending on the ventricular rate. If symptomatic, treatment should include atropine and a transcutaneous or transvenous pacemaker. A permanent pacemaker may be required if the underlying cause is not corrected.

With **third-degree heart block,** or **complete heart block,** there is no communication between the atria and ventricles; therefore the atria are completely dissociated from the ventricles. There will be P waves throughout the rhythm, but NOT associated with the QRS complexes, so the PR intervals will be variable throughout the rhythm strip. The QRS complexes may be narrow (junctional escape rhythm) or wide (idioventricular rhythm). Patients with this type of block are usually symptomatic, depending on the ventricular rate. If symptomatic, treatment should include atropine and a transcutaneous or transvenous pacemaker. A permanent pacemaker may be required if the underlying cause is not corrected.

17. What is atrioventricular (AV) nodal reentrant tachycardia?

AV nodal reentrant tachycardia (AVNRT) is a benign tachycardia; that is, it is not life-threatening. It can occur at any age and may cause palpitations or a sensation of pulsations in the neck, dizziness/light-headedness, weakness, or hypotension. It is usually not associated with structural heart disease. Within the AV node there are actually two conduction pathways, a slow pathway (alpha) and a fast pathway (beta). These pathways have different conduction velocities and different refractory periods. They share one final common pathway through the lower part of the AV node and the bundle of His. In sinus rhythm, the electrical impulse travels down the fast pathway to depolarize the ventricles. The impulse also travels down the slow pathway, but terminates there because the final common pathway is refractory when the impulse reaches it.

Because there are two different electrical pathways within the AV node with two different conduction velocities and two different refractory periods, the stage is set for reentry. The slow pathway has a short refractory period and therefore recovers before the fast pathway. If a premature atrial complex (PAC) occurs at the moment when the fast pathway is still refractory, the impulse travels down the slow pathway and then retrograde over the fast pathway, which is no longer refractory when the impulse reaches it. Therefore a reentry circuit is created. This type of reentry is called the "slow-fast" reentry circuit and is found in about 90% of patients with AVNRT. The remaining 10% of patients have a "fast-slow" reentry circuit, where the tachycardia is initiated by a premature ventricular contraction and the impulse travels retrograde over the slow pathway. This is an uncommon form of AVNRT.

During sinus rhythm the ECG is normal, but during tachycardia the rhythm is regular (rate 150 to 250 beats per minute [beats/min]) with a narrow QRS complex. Since there is retrograde conduction to the atria, there will be inverted P waves in leads II, III, and aV_F. However, when the rate is this fast, the P waves are often buried in the QRS complex and may not be identified. Sometimes the P wave may distort the end of the QRS complex.

18. What is the treatment for AVNRT?

The treatment for AVNRT consists of medications such as calcium blockers or beta-blockers; however, the side effects may not be tolerable. Radiofrequency ablation of the slow pathway in many cases provides a cure for this arrhythmia.

19. What is Wolff-Parkinson-White syndrome?

Wolff-Parkinson-White (WPW) syndrome is a type of preexcitation syndrome. Preexcitation occurs when the ventricular myocardium is activated by an atrial impulse earlier than expected because of a congenital extra electrical connection between the atria and ventricles not attached to the normal conduction system. WPW syndrome includes several classic ECG findings and is often associated with atrioventricular reentrant tachycardias. Patients may exhibit symptoms at any time; usually the chief complaint is palpitations that can be controlled using vagal maneuvers.

In WPW syndrome the accessory pathway, called the bundle of Kent, connects the atria directly to the ventricles. The pathway can be located anywhere around the atrioventricular groove. In a small number of patients, there may be more than one accessory pathway. This accessory pathway sets up the reentry circuit with the AV node, both of which may be capable of antegrade (down) and retrograde (up) conduction. This may cause narrow or wide complex tachycardias. The tachycardias will be wide when impulses are conducted antegrade over the accessory pathway and retrograde through the AV node. The tachycardias will be narrow when the impulses are conducted antegrade through the AV node and retrograde over the accessory pathway.

When the patient is in sinus rhythm, some of the atrial impulse travels over the accessory pathway, which does not have the normal delay of the AV node, creating a P wave with a short PR interval. When the impulse reaches the ventricles, which occurs in less than 0.12 second, the electrical impulse is outside the specialized Purkinje fibers. This causes ventricular depolarization, which occurs slowly at first, creating the characteristic delta wave (a slurring of the early portion of the R wave). Since some of the sinus impulse also travels through the AV node, the remainder of the ventricular depolarization occurs via the Purkinje system, so the rest of the QRS complex looks normal.

20. What is the difference between orthodromic atrioventricular (AV) reentrant tachycardia and antidromic AV reentrant tachycardia in WPW syndrome?

Orthodromic AV reentrant tachycardia accounts for the majority of tachycardias in WPW syndrome. It is initiated by a premature atrial contraction conducted antegrade (down) over the AV node to the ventricles and then retrograde (up) over the accessory pathway, stimulating the atria. It then travels back down the AV node again and up the accessory pathway, continually repeating this "circus movement tachycardia." Because the impulse travels down the AV node, the tachycardia will have regular and narrow QRS complexes. P waves usually follow the QRS complexes, and the delta wave is not seen since the entire electrical impulse travels down the AV node.

Antidromic AV reentrant tachycardia is less common than orthodromic AV reentrant tachycardia. It only occurs in about 10% of patients with WPW syndrome. In this case, the premature atrial contraction travels antegrade (down) through the accessory pathway into the ventricles outside the Purkinje system, creating regular, wide, bizarre QRS complexes with delta waves. It then travels retrograde (up) through the AV node, depolarizing the atria, and then back down the accessory pathway, up the AV node; this is repeated continually, creating a reentrant wide complex tachycardia.

21. How is WPW syndrome treated?

The reentrant tachycardias of WPW syndrome can be treated with medications, although WPW syndrome can be successfully cured with an electrophysiology study to isolate the accessory pathway followed by radiofrequency ablation to destroy the pathway.

22. Why is atrial fibrillation dangerous in a patient with WPW syndrome?

Patients who have atrial fibrillation without an accessory pathway are not in danger of the life-threatening arrhythmia ventricular fibrillation because the AV node protects the ventricle from high atrial rates as a result of its inherent property to delay impulses as they pass through the AV node. When there is an accessory pathway present that is capable of antegrade conduction and a patient develops atrial fibrillation, the QRS complexes will be irregular as well as wide and bizarre with a delta wave, depending on how much of the electrical impulse is conducted down the accessory pathway and how much is conducted down the AV node. The accessory pathway does not have the property of slowing electrical impulses; therefore if the accessory pathway is the sole propagator of the impulse, potentially each of the 350 to 600 electrical impulses in the atria can be conducted down to the ventricles in a 1:1 fashion, causing ventricular fibrillation.

When a patient with known WPW syndrome develops atrial fibrillation, AV node blocking drugs (for example, digitalis, beta-blockers, and calcium blockers) should not be given, as these medications will potentially cause hypotension and may enhance conduction down the accessory pathway, making a bad situation worse. If the patient is hemodynamically unstable, synchronized cardioversion is the treatment of choice.

23. What is the differential diagnosis of wide complex tachycardia?

- Ventricular tachycardia (VT)
- Supraventricular tachycardia (SVT) with antegrade conduction over an accessory pathway (Wolff-Parkinson-White syndrome)
- Aberrant conduction

- Supraventricular tachycardia
- Upper rate limit ventricular pacing (with small pacemaker artifacts)

24. How are antiarrhythmic drugs classified?

Antiarrhythmic drugs are classified according to their effect on the action potential. The Vaughn-Williams classification, developed in 1975, has been the most widely used classification system.

Antiarrhythmic drugs

Class	Examples	Inotropic Effect
I Membrane stabilizers (fast channel sodium blockers)	IA: Quinidine Procainamide Disopyramide	Negative
	IB: Lidocaine Tocainide Mexiletine Phenytoin	No effect
	IC: Flecainide Encainide Morcizine Propafenone	Negative
II Beta blockers	Metoprolol Atenolol Many others	Negative Negative Negative
III Neural adrenergic agonists	Bretylium Amiodarone Sotalol Dofetilide Ibutilide	No effect No effect Negative No effect No effect
IV Slow channel calcium agonists	Verapamil Diltiazem	Negative Negative

Data from Huszar RJ: *Basic dysrhythmias: interpretation and management*, St Louis, 2002, Mosby.

25. Why are isolated premature ventricular contractions not treated with oral medications in post myocardial infarction (MI) patients in order to prevent progression to a life-threatening arrhythmia?

The Cardiac Arrhythmia Suppression Trial (CAST) in the late 1980s studied suppression of premature ventricular contractions (PVCs) in post myocardial infarction (MI) patients with oral antiarrhythmic drugs. Historically, post MI

PVCs were thought to be a precursor of more life-threatening arrhythmias. The patients studied in the CAST trial were asymptomatic or mildly symptomatic and had left ventricular ejection fractions <40%. The study was terminated prematurely when it was identified that there was an increase in morbidity (all cause sudden death) in those patients treated with antiarrhythmic medications, specifically encainide and flecainide, both class IC agents. This was attributed to the drugs' "proarrhythmic" effect, which is the ability of a drug to worsen the arrhythmia it is used to treat. This study drastically changed the way ventricular arrhythmias are treated in post MI patients and in patients with coronary artery disease.

26. **Why have we seen an increase in the use of implantable cardioverter-defibrillators (ICDs)?**

Before 2002 patients could only receive an ICD if they had nonsustained VT and were inducible during electrophysiology (EP) testing or if they sustained a witnessed cardiac arrest. Results from the Multicenter Automatic Defibrillator Implantation Trial II (MADIT II), published in 2002, looked at prophylactic implantation of a defibrillator in 1232 patients with a history of an MI and reduced left ventricular ejection fractions (≤30%). These patients did not undergo EP testing to determine induciblity. The researchers found that prophylactic implantation of a defibrillator resulted in improved survival in these patients.

27. **If a patient requires antiarrhythmic therapy in addition to an implantable defibrillator because of recurrent VT, what are the drugs of choice?**

The most commonly prescribed oral medications for VT are the class III oral antiarrhythmics. The class I drugs are rarely used because of their proarrhythmic effects.

28. **What is the difference between idioventricular rhythm, accelerated idioventricular rhythm, and ventricular tachycardia, and how are they treated?**

Idioventricular rhythm, also referred to as ventricular escape rhythm, occurs when higher pacemakers in the heart (the atria and the AV node) fail. The inherent firing rate of the ventricles is <40 beats/min. There will be three or more QRS complexes in a row, and they will be wide and bizarre. There will be no P waves with failure of the higher pacemakers. Treatment for this rhythm depends on the symptoms the patient is experiencing. At heart rates of 40 beats/min, the patient may have no symptoms; however, a transcutaneous pacemaker should be immediately available in case the heart rate falls and/or the patient becomes hemodynamically unstable. Atropine should be available as it may increase the sinus rate to allow the sinus node to gain control as the dominant pacemaker in the heart. The patient may need a temporary pacemaker if the rhythm is sustained. This rhythm should not be treated with antiarrhythmics because these drugs may obliterate the ventricular rhythm and cause asystole if there is truly failure of higher pacemakers. Investigation should include reasons for failure of higher pacemakers (for example, medications, complete AV block, advanced heart disease).

Accelerated idioventricular rhythm (AIVR) occurs when there are three or more consecutive ventricular beats with a rate between 40 and 100 beats/min. The term "slow VT" has been used to identify this rhythm; however, it is an inappropriate term. AIVR may be seen in the setting of an acute MI and is usually self-limiting. Since the rate of AIVR is often close to the sinus rate, patients are usually asymptomatic. Additionally, it is not unusual to see fusion beats (a QRS complex that looks like a combination of the pure sinus QRS complex and the pure ventricular complex) at the beginning and end of the run of AIVR since the sinus and ventricular rates are close. AIVR occurs when the ventricular rate becomes faster than the sinus rate or if the sinus rate slows. The appearance of fusion beats confirms the wide, bizarre rhythm is ventricular in origin. AIVR is not usually associated with hemodynamic compromise and is usually transient. Treatment may include the use of atropine or atrial pacing if the AV dissociation causes hemodynamic compromise.

Ventricular tachycardia (VT) consists of three or more consecutive ventricular beats with a rate of >100 beats/min. It is often seen in patients with an acute or prior myocardial infarction, coronary artery disease, and dilated cardiomyopathy. If the patient is stable with an ejection fraction of >40%, medications such as IV procainamide, amiodarone, or lidocaine may be used. If there is a low ejection fraction (<40%), then amiodarone is the first choice. Lidocaine may also be used. Synchronized cardioversion may be performed at any time, assuming the patient is well sedated before cardioversion. If the patient is unstable, then proceed directly to synchronized cardioversion.

29. What is the difference between monomorphic ventricular tachycardia and polymorphic ventricular tachycardia?

Monomorphic ventricular tachycardia is identified when each of the QRS complexes has an identical or nearly identical morphology. Polymorphic ventricular tachycardia exists when the morphology of the QRS complexes changes from beat to beat during the tachycardia.

30. What is torsades de pointe and how is it managed?

A subset of polymorphic ventricular tachycardia is an arrhythmia called torsades de pointe; this occurs when there are changes in the QRS complex polarity creating the appearance that the QRS's are rotating around the baseline. Torsades de pointe is usually associated with a prolonged QT interval, either inherited or acquired. The inherited form is referred to as idiopathic long QT syndrome. It is usually treated with beta-blockers and a pacemaker/ICD.

Other causes of acquired QT prolongation, which may lead to polymorphic ventricular tachycardia or torsades de pointe, include electrolyte abnormalities (hypokalemia, hypomagnesemia, and hypocalcemia), high-protein liquid diets, or severe coronary ischemia.

Treatment of polymorphous VT includes discontinuation of the offending drugs or correction of the underlying abnormality. IV magnesium is used for more immediate treatment (bolus followed by a continuous infusion).

31. What are the most common reasons for acquired prolonged QT intervals?

Medication use is the most common reason for acquired prolonged QT intervals. These medications may include:

- Class IA antiarrhythmics along with sotalol and amiodarone (the most common offenders)
- Psychotropic drugs (for example, tricyclic antidepressants and phenothiazines)
- Antihistamines (for example, terfenadine [Seldane] and astemizole [Hismanal])
- Antibiotics (erythromycin, pentamidine, ampicillin)
- Miscellaneous drugs (probucol, ketanserin, cocaine, papaverine)

32. How do you correct the QT interval?

It is important to calculate the measured QT interval (QTm) and then to correct the QT interval (QTc) for the patient's heart rate. The calculation used to correct the QT interval for the patient's heart rate is:

$$QTc = \frac{QTm}{\sqrt{R\text{-to-R interval (in seconds)}}}$$

33. Why is it important to be able to differentiate between ventricular tachycardia (VT) and supraventricular tachycardia (SVT) that is aberrantly conducted?

One of the most common mistakes made by health care providers is to consider the diagnosis of VT *unlikely* when the arrhythmia is hemodynamically well tolerated. The diagnosis of VT should be high on the differential list until proven otherwise. It is important to be able to distinguish between the types of wide complex tachycardias because one medication commonly used to treat SVT, verapamil, can cause severe hemodynamic deterioration in patients with true VT. Additionally, medications used to treat VT, amiodarone and procainamide, may be withheld for a prolonged period while the patient is being treated for what is presumed to be SVT.

According to advanced cardiac life support (ACLS) guidelines, if the patient is hemodynamically stable with a wide complex tachycardia, obtain a 12-lead ECG, if possible. If unable to confirm the wide complex tachycardia as SVT or VT using either the ECG or the physical findings, then attempt to identify if the patient has preserved cardiac function or if the patient has an ejection fraction ≤40% or congestive heart failure (CHF). If the patient has preserved cardiac function, then use procainamide, amiodarone, or synchronized cardioversion. If the patient has an ejection fraction ≤40% or CHF, use amiodarone or synchronized cardioversion. Remember to sedate your patient before using synchronized cardioversion.

If the patient with a wide complex tachycardia is unstable, then the immediate treatment is synchronized cardioversion.

34. **What are the basic electrocardiographic features used to determine if a wide complex tachycardia is ventricular in nature or supraventricular in nature?**

A 12-lead ECG is very helpful when trying to determine the cause of a wide complex tachycardia; therefore one should be obtained if time is available. The four basic criteria used to distinguish between ventricular tachycardia (VT) and supraventricular tachycardia (SVT) with aberration are atrioventricular (AV) dissociation, QRS width, QRS axis, and morphology of the QRS complex in V_1 and V_6.

Identification of AV dissociation during tachycardia strongly favors the diagnosis of VT; however, failure to observe AV dissociation does not mean the rhythm should be interpreted as SVT with aberration. The presence of fusion or capture beats may help identify AV dissociation. If the patient has epicardial wires after heart surgery, an atrial electrogram may help identify AV dissociation. Physical signs of AV dissociation include the following: cannon alpha wave in the neck, changing intensity of S_1, and beat-to-beat changes in systolic blood pressure.

A QRS width greater than 0.14 seconds strongly favors VT, but the QRS width should be confirmed in more than one lead, if possible. Care must be taken using this criterion if the patient has a preexisting bundle branch block, an accessory pathway with antegrade conduction over the pathway, or digoxin toxicity.

A QRS axis in the "northwest" quadrant, also referred to as the indeterminate axis or "no man's land" axis, is strongly indicative of VT. A left axis deviation with a mainly **positive QRS** in V_1 is often found with VT. However, a left axis deviation with a mainly negative QRS deflection in V_1 is of **no** prognostic value. A normal axis or right axis deviation is more common in SVT with aberration.

QRS morphology in V_1 and V_6 can be useful to identify the type of wide complex tachycardia. When the QRS is mainly positive in V_1 (similar to a right bundle branch block configuration), then the following clues will be helpful: If there is a monophasic or biphasic QRS pattern in V_1 or a QRS with "rabbit ears" where the **left** "rabbit ear" is **taller** than the right "rabbit ear", then the wide complex tachycardia is probably VT. Additionally, if the R/S ratio in V_6 is <1, the diagnosis favors VT. However, if there is a triphasic RSR in V_1 or a QRS pattern in V_1, then the diagnosis favors SVT with aberration.

When the QRS is mainly negative in V_1 (similar to a left bundle branch configuration), then the following clues will be helpful. If the R wave in V_1 or V_2 is >40 milliseconds or if there is a notched or "slurred" downstroke of the S wave in V_1 or V_2, the diagnosis favors VT. Additionally, if there is >60 milliseconds from the R wave to the nadir of the S wave or if there is any Q in V_6, the diagnosis favors VT. However, if there is a narrow R wave (<40 milliseconds) and/or a clean downstroke of the S wave in V_1 **or** V_2, the diagnosis favors SVT with aberration.

Another clue to help identify a wide complex tachycardia as VT is concordance in the V leads (where all the QRS complexes in the V leads are either all positively deflected or all negatively deflected). If the patient has a history of nonsustained VT or PVCs, a history of a myocardial infarction, decreased left ventricular function, or a left ventricular aneurysm, the diagnosis of VT is also favored.

35. What is new in the ACLS algorithm for pulseless ventricular tachycardia (VT) and ventricular fibrillation (VF)?

After verifying unresponsiveness and establishing the airway, breathing, and circulation, defibrillation is still the first treatment for pulseless VT or VF, after verification of the rhythm. First defibrillate with 200 joules (J), then with 200 to 300 J, and then with 360 J (or equivalent biphasic), if necessary.

If defibrillation is unsuccessful, then a vasopressor such as epinephrine or vasopressin should be administered. Epinephrine is administered as a 1-milligram (mg) IV bolus, followed by a 20-milliliter (ml) flush of IV fluid. This should be repeated every 3 to 5 minutes during resuscitation and followed each time by defibrillation with 360 J (or equivalent biphasic). If there is no IV line available, epinephrine may be administered via the endotracheal tube (2.0 to 2.5 mg in 10 ml of normal saline). Vasopressin is a new drug in the armamentarium for pulseless VT and VF. It may be substituted for epinephrine. Vasopressin is a potent vasoconstrictor. It is unlikely to cause beta stimulation and postarrest adrenergic storm. It is administered as a single dose of 40 units IV followed by a 20-ml flush of IV fluid. Within 30 to 60 seconds after the dose, the patient should be defibrillated with 360 J (or equivalent biphasic). If necessary, within 5 to 10 minutes after the vasopressin dose, consider using epinephrine as described above (vasopressin is only given once).

If attempts to restore a rhythm remain unsuccessful, then consider the use of antiarrhythmics in the following order: amiodarone and lidocaine. Additionally, consider the use of magnesium if the patient is known to be hypomagnesemic. If needed, resume attempts to defibrillate.

Key Points

- Atrial fibrillation is referred to as paroxysmal, persistent, or chronic.
- Intravenous magnesium is the treatment of choice for torsades de pointes.
- Patients should be monitored in lead V_1 for arrhythmias.

Internet Resources

National Heart, Lung, and Blood Institute: Arrhythmias:
http://www.nlm.nih.gov/medlineplus/ency/article001101.html

The New England Journal of Medicine:
http://www.nejm.org/cgi/collection/arrhythmias

Bibliography

Andries E, Brugada P, Brugada J, Steurer G, Podrid PJ: A practical approach to the diagnosis of a tachycardia with a wide QRS complex. In Podrid PJ, Kowey PR, editors: *Cardiac Arrhythmia: Mechanisms, Diagnosis, and Management*, Baltimore, 1995, Williams & Wilkins.

Brzozowski LA: Wide QRS complex tachycardia, *AACN Clin Iss* 3(1):173-179, 1992.

Bubien RS, Sanchez JE: Atrial fibrillation: treatment rationale and clinical utility of nonpharmacologic therapies, *AACN Clin Iss* 12(1):140-155, 2001.

Cain ME: Atrial fibrillation—rhythm or rate control, *N Engl J Med* 347(23):1822-1823, 2002.

Conover MB: *Understanding electrocardiography*, St Louis, 2003, Mosby.

Esberger D, Jones S, Morris F: Clinical review. ABC of clinical electrocardiography: junctional tachycardias, *Br Med J* 324(7338):662-665, 2002.

Fuster V, Rydén LE, Asinger RW, Cannom DS, Crijns HJ, Frye RL, Halpern JL, Kay GN, Klein WW, Lévy S, McNamara RL, Prystowsky EN, Wann LS, Wyse DG: ACC/AHA/ESC guidelines for the management of patients with atrial fibrillation: executive summary: a report of the American College of Cardiology/American Heart Association Task Force on Practice Guidelines and the European Society of Cardiology Committee for Practice Guidelines and Policy Conferences (Committee to Develop Guidelines for the Management of Patients with Atrial Fibrillation), *Circulation* 104:2118-2150, 2001.

Housholder-Hughes SD: Advanced cardiac life support for the new millennium, *J Cardiovasc Nurs* 16(3): 9-23, 87-88, 2002.

Huszar RJ: *Basic dysrhythmias: interpretation and management*, St Louis, 2002, Mosby.

Kantachuvessiri A: Pulmonary veins: preferred site for catheter ablation of atrial fibrillation, *Heart Lung: J Acute Crit Care* 31(4):271-278, 2002.

Kern KB, Halperin HR, Field J: Contempo updates: linking evidence and experience. New guidelines for cardiopulmonary resuscitation and emergency cardiac care: changes in the management of cardiac arrest, *JAMA* 285(10):1267-1269, 1373-1374, 2001.

Moss AJ, Zareba W, Hall WJ, Klein H, Wilber DJ, Cannom DS, Daubert JP, Higgins SL, Brown MW, Andrews ML: Multicenter automatic defibrillator implantation trial II investigators. Prophylactic implantation of a defibrillator in patients with myocardial infarction and reduced ejection fraction, *N Engl J Med* 346(12):877-883, 2002.

Oral H, Knight BP, Tada H, et al: Pulmonary vein isolation for paroxysmal and persistent atrial fibrillation, *Circulation* 105:1077-1081, 2002.

Van Gelder IC, Hagens VE, Bosker HA, Kingma JH, Kamp O, Kingma T, Said SA, Darmanata JI, Timmermans AJM, Tijssen JGP, Crijns HJG: A comparison of rate control and rhythm control in patients with atrial fibrillation, *N Engl J Med* 347(23):1825-1833, 2002.

Van Gelder IC, Hagens VE, Bosker HA, Kingma JH, Kamp O, Kingma T, Said SA, Darmanata JI, Timmermans AJM, Tijssen JGP, Crijns HJG: A comparison of rate control and rhythm control in patients with recurrent persistent atrial fibrillation, *N Engl J Med* 347(23):1834-1840, 2002.

Chapter 9

Cardiomyopathy

Donna Chojnowski

1. Define and classify cardiomyopathy.

Cardiomyopathy (CM) is a term that designates heart disease that directly involves the myocardium, excluding pericardial, valvular, and ischemic disease. The most widely accepted classification system is one used by the World Health Organization and the International Society and Federation of Cardiology. This classification system recognizes and classifies CM by specific pathophysiological characteristics. The basic functional classes identified include *dilated, hypertrophic,* and *restrictive* cardiomyopathy. Additional classifications include *arrhythmogenic right ventricular* CM and *unclassified* CM. Primary CM refers to diseases that only involve the myocardium and in which the disease process is not known or is not a manifestation of a systemic disease. Secondary CM, however, includes cardiomyopathy that is a result of another cardiovascular disorder or systemic disease.

2. Define dilated cardiomyopathy (DCM).

Dilated CM (DCM) involves ventricular dilatation with contractile dysfunction that progressively leads to heart failure symptomatology. DCM accounts for 60% of all diagnosed cardiomyopathy.

3. Define hypertrophic cardiomyopathy.

Hypertrophic CM (HCM) involves excessive hypertrophy of the left ventricle. The hypertrophy is usually asymmetrical and often involves the interventricular septum. The location of the septal hypertrophy can result in obstructive interference with ventricular outflow. Hyperdynamic ventricular function is present until the disease process advances.

4. Define restrictive cardiomyopathy.

Restrictive CM (RCM) is less common in Western countries and is characterized by stiff ventricles and impaired diastolic function.

5. Describe arrhythmogenic right ventricular cardiomyopathy.

Arrhythmogenic right ventricular CM (formerly RV dysplasia) involves the loss of myocardial cells in the right ventricle and is associated with reentrant ventricular tachyarrhythmias.

6. What is unclassified cardiomyopathy?

Unclassified CM is the category of fibroelastosis disorders that leads to systolic dysfunction secondary to thickening of the left ventricular endocardium from growth of fibrous and elastic tissue.

7. What is the etiology and clinical course for dilated cardiomyopathy (DCM)?

There are more than 75 specific diseases of the heart muscle that lead to the characteristics of DCM with the resulting dilated ventricles and contractile dysfunction. This decreased contractile function triggers a series of complex neurohormonal responses that initially are compensatory, but become counterproductive, contributing to the onset of heart failure. A significant number of DCM patients have an unclear etiology and are diagnosed as idiopathic. There are certain mechanisms suspected to influence this disorder, including familial influences, genetic factors, viral infections, unidentified cytotoxins, and immunologic abnormalities. Of note, familial CM is diagnosed most often; 20% of persons identified with idiopathic CM have been found to have a first-degree relative that has been diagnosed with DCM.

Idiopathic DCM accounts for 25% of heart failure cases in the United States, with the remaining 75% of cases being the result of hypertension and coronary disease.

The natural history process of DCM is not clear. Many patients have minimal or absent symptoms during the disease progression for months to years.

It is still difficult to predict the clinical course because there is no reliability for prediction with any one indicator. The prognosis is clearly graver for the person diagnosed with advanced dilated biventricular enlargement and worsened contractile function.

8. Describe the new classification of heart failure (HF).

New classification of heart failure

Stage	Definition
Stage A	No diagnosed structural heart disease, but have risk factors that can lead to heart failure
Stage B	History of structural heart disease, but may be asymptomatic
Stage C	Patients with structural heart disease and current or prior history of heart failure symptoms
Stage D	Patients with refractory end-stage heart

From Hunt SA, et al: ACC/AHA guidelines for the evaluation and management of chronic heart failure in the adult: A report of the American College of Cardiology/American Heart Association Task Force on Practice Guidelines (Committee to Revise the 1995 Guidelines for the Evaluation and Management of Heart Failure), 2001. Available at: http://www.acc.org/clinical/guidelines/failure/hf_index.html.

9. How is DCM diagnosed?

The patient with DCM may initially be asymptomatic with gradual occurrence of symptoms; the most common complaints are fatigue, weakness, and dyspnea. As the disease progresses, additional symptoms include, but are not limited to, chest pain, palpitations, cough, abdominal bloating, nausea and vomiting, and anorexia.

Identification of the disease as DCM requires a thorough history and physical examination in conjunction with diagnostic studies.

10. What factors should be included when taking the patient's history?

- Onset of symptoms
- Quality of symptoms
- Associated symptoms
- Relieving factors
- Medication and diet history
- Social history: alcohol use, cigarette smoking, and illicit drug use
- Family history

11. What should the review of symptoms (ROS) include?

Neurology: depression, syncope, confusion, difficulty with concentration, anxiety, panic attacks, cerebral vascular disease, seizures

Cardiovascular: angina, nonspecific chest pain, fatigue, orthostasis, palpitations, edema, temperature changes in extremities, discoloration in extremities, coronary disease, hyperlipidemia, hypertension

Pulmonary: dyspnea at rest or with exertion, cough, orthopnea, paroxysmal nocturnal dyspnea, hemoptysis, wheezing, asthma, lung disease, pulmonary emboli, pneumonia, sleep apnea

Gastroenterology: abdominal bloating, nausea, vomiting, anorexia, weight loss or gain, stool patterns, gastritis, gastroesophageal reflux

Genitourinary: nocturia, oliguria, anuria, nephrolithiasis, renal insufficiency, urinary tract infections, sexually transmitted diseases

Endocrine: history of thyroid disease; changes in skin, hair, or temperature preference; diabetes

12. What are the usual physical examination findings?

Usual physical examination findings

Parameter	Finding
Blood pressure	Normal or hypotensive, narrow pulse pressure
Heart rate	Tachycardia, regular or irregular
Respirations	Tachypneic on exertion
Mental status	Disorientation
Skin	Cyanosis, edema
Neck veins	Distended
Heart	Diffuse apical impulse, ventricular heave or lift, third or fourth heart sound; murmur of tricuspid and/or mitral regurgitation
Lungs	Clear to crackles; decreased tactile fremitus
Abdomen	Ascites, enlarged liver span; elevated hepatojugular reflex
Extremities	Edema

13. What diagnostic tests are indicated?

Lab work: Basic biochemical lab work is done to evaluate the patient's general condition and any systemic effects. Routine labs evaluate renal function, metabolic imbalance, and anemia. Additional lab work may include testing for thyroid disease, hemochromatosis, hypocalcemia, HIV, uremia, and drug levels.

Chest x-ray: The chest x-ray evaluates the cardiothoracic ratio and shows cardiomegaly and the presence of pulmonary vascular congestion and interstitial edema. A pleural effusion may also be noted.

Electrocardiogram: The ECG usually shows tachycardia; the presence of atrial and/or ventricular arrhythmias is common. Poor R wave progression and intraventricular conduction abnormalities such as left bundle branch block may be noted. There may be evidence of ischemic heart disease. Of note, patients with DCM may have Q waves and nonspecific ST-T wave abnormalities because of significant ventricular fibrosis.

Echocardiogram: Two-dimensional and Doppler forms of the echocardiogram can provide a significant amount of information about the patient with DCM.

This procedure evaluates the chambers, valves, pericardium, myocardium, and global function. Specific information about the chamber size and shape, systolic wall thickening, fractional shortening of ventricles, wall motion analysis, valve integrity and motion, and presence of pericardial effusion or restriction can be identified.

Additional testing: This may include a combination of studies to further evaluate the patient, confirm the diagnosis, and determine the treatment regimen. Testing may include cardiac catheterization, endomyocardial biopsy, hemodynamic assessment, radionuclide ventriculography, cardiopulmonary exercise testing with oxygen consumption (VO_2), magnetic resonance imaging (MRI), and computed tomography (CT). After the initial diagnostic workup and treatment, the studies continued for ongoing evaluation of therapy usually include patient examinations with interview, echocardiography, ECG, and VO_2 exercise testing. In advanced disease states, hemodynamic assessment will be important for therapy adjustment.

14. What hemodynamic patterns are common for DCM?

Left and right heart catheterization usually shows elevated left ventricular end-diastolic pressure (LVEDP) and elevated pulmonary capillary wedge pressure (PCWP). As the disease advances and left ventricular function deteriorates, cardiac output and cardiac index will decrease concomitant with an increase in pulmonary artery and pulmonary capillary wedge pressures. As the declining cardiac output and cardiac index become unable to meet the metabolic demands for oxygen consumption, there will also be a significant decrease in mixed venous oxygen saturation (MVO_2). In the setting of mitral regurgitation, the presence of an enlarged v wave will be noted on PAP and PCW tracings. If the right ventricular function is also affected, there will be an elevation in right atrial (RA) and right ventricular (RV) pressures.

15. Discuss treatment options for patients with DCM.

The disease progression of DCM leads to heart failure (HF) as a result of the remodeling process that occurs. Patients with an identified specific disorder leading to DCM will have treatment directed at elimination and/or control of the underlying disease, unlike idiopathic DCM where there is no specific therapy. All patients with DCM will rely on HF management to retard the progression of the disease and symptoms. Remodeling is a progressive process by which mechanical, neurohormonal, and possibly genetic factors alter the configuration and function of the left ventricle. The configuration of the ventricle changes by dilatation, hypertrophy, and becoming more spherical in shape.

16. What is anaerobic threshold?

Anaerobic threshold is the point when the metabolic demands are not met and muscle tissues convert to anaerobic metabolism for energy. The anaerobic threshold level is reduced in patients with heart failure.

17. What is cardiopulmonary exercise testing for oxygen consumption (VO₂)?

Cardiopulmonary VO_2 exercise testing involves exercising a patient on a treadmill or stationary bicycle while simultaneously monitoring their vital signs, ECG results, airflow, and respiratory gas exchange. These measurements are then used to determine maximal oxygen consumption and anaerobic threshold, thereby predicting cardiac reserve. VO_2 results greater than 20 ml/min/kg signify mild to no functional impairment, results in the range 10 to 16 ml/min/kg indicate moderate to severe impairment, and VO_2 measurements less than 6 ml/min/kg represent very severe impairment. VO_2 testing is a diagnostic tool used to determine a patient's functional capability and is an adjunct in the evaluation of the seriousness of the cardiac disease. Repeat VO_2 testing is used to follow the disease progression and to evaluate the patient's response to therapy.

18. Describe arrhythmogenic right ventricular cardiomyopathy (ARVD).

This unusual cardiomyopathy is also known as right ventricular dysplasia. In ARVD myocardial cells of the right ventricle are lost and then replaced with adipose and fibrous tissue. There is a genetic link in at least one third of the cases of ARVD, and ARVD is found predominantly in males. This diagnosis is made based on a combination of clinical and diagnostic findings. The most common reported symptoms are palpitations and syncope. There is a risk of sudden death associated with ventricular fibrillation.

19. What are the clinical findings in patients with ARVD?

The physical exam usually is unremarkable unless left ventricular dysfunction is present. The ECG findings may show inverted T waves in the right precordial leads, left bundle branch block, and arrhythmias. Electrophysiological studies often show evidence of reentrant ventricular tachyarrhythmias originating from the right ventricle. An echocardiogram shows a dilated and poorly contracting right ventricle and usually a normal left ventricle. MRI testing has also been used to identify this disorder.

20. What is the treatment for ARVD?

Treatment for ARVD includes primarily antiarrhythmic therapy, especially beta-blockers, sotalol, and amiodarone. There has been success with radiofrequency ablation and internal cardiac defibrillators (ICDs). Refractory cases are considered for heart transplant.

21. Explain the incidence and pathophysiology of hypertrophic cardiomyopathy (HCM).

Primary hypertrophic cardiomyopathy is identified as myocardial hypertrophy without a secondary cause such as hypertension; the hypertrophy is usually asymmetrical and involves the septal wall of the left ventricle. The ventricular systolic function is hyperdynamic and sometimes associated with a dynamic left ventricular outflow gradient. Histologically, there is cellular and myofiber disarray with myocardial fibrosis, and medial intimal proliferation of small coronary arteries. HCM was previously known by the term idiopathic hypertrophic subaortic stenosis.

This disorder is found in approximately 0.2% of the general population. There is a genetic association identified as familial HCM that has been considered genetically heterogeneous because of the identification of several genes and mutations linking the disorder. The majority of patients at the time of diagnosis with HCM are asymptomatic or are mildly short of breath, and they are diagnosed with HCM after their history reveals a family member with the diagnosis of HCM. Other individuals are diagnosed at necropsy after sudden death.

The disease is often identified in the 30- to 40-year age group and is slightly more common in males. In children the early diagnosis of HCM is important because of a higher mortality from sudden death. This disorder has been diagnosed in the elderly population but is challenging because of aging factors.

The most significant physiological feature of HCM is the ventricular hypertrophy with or without the outflow gradient. This hypertrophy and myocardial cellular fibrosis lead to diastolic dysfunction because of left ventricular stiffness that impairs diastolic relaxation and ventricular filling. The increased LVEDP from this diastolic impairment causes pulmonary congestion and dyspnea in spite of the hyperdynamic systolic function and cardiac output.

Another feature of HCM is the left ventricular outflow gradient that is present in some patients. This pressure gradient is related to the hypertophied septal wall, the hyperdynamic activity of the left ventricle in systole, and the systolic anterior motion of the mitral valve leaflet. The gradient develops as the blood flows from the left ventricle through the outflow tract to the aorta in a narrowed area that is further hampered by the anterior movement of the mitral valve leaflet causing obstruction. This pressure gradient or obstruction is dynamic and influenced by maneuvers that alter preload and afterload. The pressure gradient changes can be identified by auscultation of a systolic murmur that intensifies with physical maneuvers that increase or decrease the pressure gradient.

The third notable feature in HCM is the development of myocardial ischemia, which can result from many factors: decreased coronary circulation secondary to outflow obstruction, hypertrophied myocardium, narrowed intramural coronaries, and increased myocardial oxygen consumption.

As the disease advances, the left ventricle dilates and contractile dysfunction occurs, leading to intractable symptoms of HF.

22. What are the clinical features associated with HCM?

The most common symptom is dyspnea from exertion. Other complaints include angina, palpitations, syncope, fatigue, paroxysmal nocturnal dyspnea, and dizziness. Physical examination shows a strong, forceful apical impulse on palpation that may be displaced laterally. The carotid pulse will have a rapid upstroke, and S_4 heart sounds will be heard. If an outflow gradient is present, the hallmark systolic murmur will be heard at the left sternal border fourth intercostal space. This murmur is harsh with a crescendo-decrescendo configuration and is intensified by maneuvers that increase the gradient such as the Valsalva maneuver, standing, and exercise. The gradient is decreased by squatting or using the Müller maneuver.

23. What are the ECG findings in patients with HCM?

The ECG is usually abnormal with left ventricular hypertrophy (LVH), ST-T wave abnormalities, prominent Q waves seen in the inferior and/or precordial leads, left axis deviation, and ventricular and atrial arrhythmias. In the setting of premature ventricular contractions and the presence of the outflow gradient, there is an increase in the contractility related to the beat post-extrasystole because of the increase in filling time secondary to the compensatory pause.

24. What are the echocardiogram and cardiac catherization findings in patients with HCM?

The echocardiogram continues to be the most useful diagnostic tool in the evaluation of this disorder. The hallmark features seen on the echocardiogram are left ventricular hypertrophy usually involving the septum and anterolateral free wall, a small LV cavity, hyperdynamic systolic function, and the presence of the outflow gradient. The echocardiogram also can assess for diastolic dysfunction. Other noninvasive testing may include an MRI and thallium imaging.

Cardiac catheterization is pursued if there is a question of coronary artery disease, but otherwise it is not necessary for diagnosis because the noninvasive echocardiogram provides sufficient information for diagnosis and evaluation. Hemodynamics, if a right heart catheterization is performed, will show pulmonary hypertension that in some cases will be moderate to severe despite an excellent cardiac output and cardiac index. The pulmonary pressures, including PCWP, will increase with exertion because of the diastolic dysfunction and elevated LVEDP.

25. Describe the treatment plan in patients with HCM.

The treatment goals for HCM are to reduce symptoms, prevent complications, and decrease the risk of sudden death. The decision to treat asymptomatic patients is not clear on the basis of available studies. Patients are ranked by assessment of risk factors such as strong family history of sudden death, syncope, cardiac arrest, ventricular arrhythmias, and significant LVH. These factors will require a more aggressive approach, which includes an ICD and amiodarone therapy. The mainstay of *drug therapy* is beta-adrenergic receptor blockers to reduce myocardial oxygen consumption, limit the heart's chronotropic response, allow for improved diastolic filling with slower heart rate, and produce an antianginal effect. Alternatives or adjuncts to beta-blocker therapy include nondihydropyridine calcium-channel antagonists, with verapamil being the most widely used. Disopyramide and diuretics are also used. Antiarrhythmic therapy for HCM is most effective when amiodarone or soltalol is used.

Patient education includes avoidance of strenuous exercise because of the risk of sudden death. The patient should thoroughly understand their diagnosis and the significance of medical therapy and follow-up. Compliance should be emphasized especially in the group of patients that is asymptomatic or has minimal symptoms.

Other treatment strategies include a dual chamber pacemaker for synchronization of the ventricles to allow for improved diastolic filling and some limited improvement in the gradient. In the setting of atrial fibrillation for the patient with HCM, an aggressive approach for conversion pharmacologically or electrically is recommended.

For the patient with significant outflow obstruction and who is refractory to medication, alternative therapies include nonsurgical reduction of the intraventricular septum or myectomy surgery with possible mitral valve replacement. Patients who require these options are in the minority, less than 5% of the total population diagnosed with HCM. Both procedures have been found to decrease the outflow gradient and improve symptom relief. The data for the surgical approach have proven long-term efficacy and more flexibility in repairing structural abnormalities. The last option for relief is cardiac transplantation, particularly in the advanced phase of the disease when the left ventricle "burns out" with dilatation and decreased function.

26. Describe the nonsurgical septal reduction for significant outflow gradients in HCM.

During cardiac catheterization an injection of ethanol into the first and sometimes second septal perforator branches of the left anterior descending artery is performed to cause a controlled myocardial infarction of the intraventricular septum, thereby decreasing the outflow gradient. The ethanol injected is 98% ethyl alcohol by volume, and the mechanism of injury is suspected to be direct injury to the cells through dehydration, resulting in tissue necrosis. Postprocedure patients may have chest pain as a result of the infarct and are treated with hydrocodone acetaminophen. Nitrates and morphine sulfate are contraindicated. Patients may require temporary pacing postprocedure, and a high complication rate of induced complete heart block requiring permanent pacemaker insertion is noted. The length of hospital stay is approximately 24 to 72 hours. The medical follow-up is within 6 weeks. The results of this procedure have demonstrated a decrease in the gradient and improved hemodynamics and functional capability by diagnostic testing.

27. Explain the incidence and pathophysiology for restrictive cardiomyopathy (RCM).

Restrictive CM is the least common in the Western world of all three major functional classes of CM. This cardiomyopathy is characterized by an impairment in diastolic filling and by ventricular rigidity due to endomyocardial and/or myocardial lesions. The systolic function usually is preserved until the disease advances. The rigidity of the ventricles causes pressure within the ventricles to rise rapidly with small increases in volume. This condition may affect either or both ventricles, leading to signs and symptoms of left-sided and/or right-sided failure because of the impaired filling. As the process advances, the ventricular cavity may become smaller, further limiting filling, because of thrombus formation on the scarred endocardium.

Endomyocardial fibrosis with or without eosinophilia is noted worldwide as the most common form of restrictive cardiomyopathy, with amyloidosis and sarcoidosis being common forms of RCM in the Western world. Less common causes include glycogen storage disease, hemochromatosis, carcinoid heart disease, and radiation. RCM can also occur without a specific known cause.

28. What are the classic symptoms associated with RCM?

The classic symptoms are fatigue, reduced exercise tolerance, and dyspnea. Patients with RCM have an inability to increase their cardiac output by tachycardia without further compromising filling. Additional symptoms noted include angina, orthopnea, paroxysmal nocturnal dyspnea, palpitations, and syncope. Some patient's symptoms initially include thromboembolic complications.

29. Describe the physical examination findings in patients with RCM.

Physical examination may show signs of right-sided heart failure such as marked fluid retention noted by increased jugular venous pressure, peripheral edema, hepatomegaly, and ascites. Kussmaul's sign, noted by an increase in jugular venous pressure on inspiration, may exist. Cardiac examination may show a palpable point of maximal impulse, which may be diffuse; the presence of heart sounds S_3, S_4, or both; and a possible systolic murmur due to atrioventricular valvular regurgitation. Vital signs may show normotensive to hypotensive blood pressure. Orthostatic hypotension may occur from overdiuresis; however, amyloid infiltration of the autonomic nervous system should be considered.

30. What diagnostic testing is used in the workup of a patient with suspected RCM?

Diagnostic testing for RCM usually requires an additional workup to diagnose the condition since constrictive pericarditis and RCM have similar clinical and hemodynamic features. The use of CT scanning, endomyocardial biopsy, and radionuclide angiography may be needed to distinguish myocardial scarring and/or infiltration from thickened pericardium.

The electrocardiogram may show sinus rhythm, supraventricular arrhythmias, or atrioventricular blocks. Low voltage may be noted. ST-segment depression or T-wave inversion may be noted in the presence of myocardial fibrosis. The echocardiogram may show a normal sized left ventricle, slightly dilated right ventricle, biatrial enlargement, thickened left ventricular wall, and pericardial effusion. The filling pattern on the echocardiogram for RCM will show an early increased left ventricular diastolic filling velocity, decreased atrial filling velocity, and decreased isovolumetric relaxation time. Advances in echocardiography are being examined and studied for effectiveness in distinguishing the diagnosis of RCM from constrictive pericarditis. The chest x-ray may be unremarkable or may show cardiomegaly because of biatrial enlargement. On x-ray pericardial calcification is absent in RCM and would be diagnostic for constrictive pericarditis.

Hemodynamics in RCM show elevated systemic and pulmonary pressures with the pulmonary systolic pressure usually greater than 50 mm Hg; however, in constrictive pericarditis the pulmonary systolic pressure is usually less than 50 mm Hg. Both disorders commonly have the characteristic dip and plateau sign otherwise known as the *square root sign*. The pattern is a deep and rapid early decline in ventricular pressure with an early diastolic dip and mid-late diastolic plateau because of the loss of ventricular distensibility. This is seen in the atrial tracing as a notable *Y* descent followed by a rapid rise and plateau. The *X* descent may also be rapid and form an M or W configuration that is also characteristic. Simultaneous measurements of left and right ventricular pressures in RCM show a difference of ≥5 mm Hg that can be enhanced with exercise, fluid challenge, or Valsalva maneuver. In constrictive pericarditis, the pressures are similar and do not change with the same maneuvers. Cardiac catheterization usually shows normal coronary anatomy, except in amyloidosis, which may have luminal irregularities.

Studies with CT and MRI will show the presence of pericardial thickening in constrictive pericarditis, not seen in RCM. The endomyocardial biopsy procedure can provide histologic information for diagnosis concerning the presence of fibrosis, scarring, and infiltration.

31. Describe treatment for RCM.

The management of RCM resulting from a specific disease includes the treatment indicated for that specific disorder. In general the treatment of RCM is directed at symptom relief and prevention of complications. As the disease advances, the response to therapy becomes more refractory. The prognosis in RCM is poor for long-term survival.

Medical therapy includes judicious administration of diuretics and ACE inhibitors. These drugs provide symptomatic benefit by decreasing venous congestion in the pulmonary and systemic circulation, and decreasing afterload. Close monitoring of these drugs is necessary, particularly during titration, because of the potential for hypotension and hypoperfusion. Lanoxin may provide some benefit and must be used with caution because of the potential for arrhythmogenicity, particularly in the setting of amyloidosis.

Because arrhythmias are common, treatment with drugs such as amiodarone and the use of internal cardiac defibrillators (ICDs) for risk of sudden death are recommended. In the setting of atrial arrhythmias such as atrial fibrillation, maintenance of sinus rhythm is essential for the atrial contribution to the cardiac output and controlled ventricular rate. Prevention of a rapid ventricular rate response is significant because of the decreased diastolic filling time that occurs, further compromising cardiac output. Fibrotic changes that occur in RCM commonly lead to conduction disease requiring permanent pacemaker therapy. Anticoagulation therapy is recommended because of the increased risk of thrombus formation in the scarred areas and the atrial appendages. Anticoagulation is also indicated for atrial fibrillation, valvular regurgitation, and decreased cardiac output.

32. **What are the goals of biventricular pacing in the treatment of heart failure?**
   - Coordinate pattern of contraction of both right and left ventricles
   - Improve heart failure symptoms by synchronizing the ventricles

 Key Points

New Classification of Heart Failure (HF):
- Stage A: No diagnosed structural heart disease, but have risk factors that can lead to heart failure
- Stage B: History of structural heart disease, but may be asymptomatic
- Stage C: Have structural heart disease and current or prior history of heart failure symptoms
- Stage D: Patients with refractory end-stage heart failure

The most common symptom associated with hypertrophic cardiomyopathy is exertional dyspnea.
The level of anaerobic threshold is reduced in heart failure.

 Internet Resources

National Heart, Lung and Blood Institute:
http://www.nhlbi.nih.gov/medlineplus/cardiomyopathy.html

Holistic Online: Cardiomyopathy:
http://www.holisticonline.com/Remedies/Heart

Bibliography

Bahler RC: Assessment of prognosis in idiopathic dilated cardiomyopathy, *Chest* 121(4):1016-1019, 2002.

Braunwald E, Zipes D, Libby P: *Heart Disease: A Textbook of Cardiovascular Medicine*, ed 6, Philadelphia, 2001, WB Saunders.

Braunwald E: Hypertrophic cardiomyopathy—the benefits of a multidisciplinary approach, *N Engl J Med* 347(17):1306-1307, 2002.

Colucci W: *Atlas of Heart Failure: Cardiac Function and Dysfunction*, ed 2, Philadelphia, 1999, Current Medicine.

Hancock EW: Differential diagnosis of restrictive cardiomyopathy and constrictive pericarditis, *Heart* 86(3):343-349, 2001.

Hunt SA, et al: ACC/AHA guidelines for the evaluation and management of chronic heart failure in the adult: A report of the American College of Cardiology/American Heart Association Task Force on Practice Guidelines (Committee to Revise the 1995 Guidelines for the Evaluation and Management of Heart Failure), 2001. Downloaded Dec 3, 2002, from the World Wide Web: http://www.acc.org/clinical/guidelines/failure/hf_index.html.

Kushwaha SS, et al: Medical progress: restrictive cardiomyopathy, *N Engl J Med* 336(4):267-276, 1997.

Lewis P: Ethanol-induced therapeutic myocardial infarction to treat hypertrophic obstructive cardiomyopathy, *Crit Care Nurs* 21(2):20-34, 2001.

Philbin E: Comprehensive multidisciplinary programs for the management of patients with congestive heart failure, *J Gen Int Med* 14:130-135, 1999.

Rajagopalan N, et al: Comparison of new Doppler echocardiographic methods to differentiate constrictive pericardial heart disease and restrictive cardiomyopthy, *Am J Cardiol* 87(1):86-94, 2001.

Shamin W, et al: Nonsurgical reduction of the interventricular septum in patients with hypertrophic cardiomyopathy, *N Engl J Med* 347(17):1326-1333, 2002.

Pericardial Disease

Kristan Devine

1. Describe the layers of the pericardium and their function.

The pericardium is comprised of two layers: visceral and parietal. The visceral pericardium is the serous layer attached to the epicardium of the heart whereas the parietal pericardium is the thick, outer layer that is rich in collagen and elastic fibers. Between these two layers lies a small amount of fluid (<50ml). The pericardium provides a physical barrier between the heart and adjacent organs, protects the heart from infection, and limits acute distention of the heart.

2. What is Beck's triad? What does it indicate?

Beck's triad is a group of three signs that are indicative of acute cardiac tamponade. These signs are:
• quiet heart sounds
• high jugular venous pressure
• low arterial pressure

3. What is pulsus paradoxus? Under what circumstances should pulsus paradoxus be assessed?

Pulsus paradoxus is a decrease in arterial blood pressure exceeding 10 mm Hg during inspiration. While pulsus paradoxus can occur because of a variety of causes, clinicians should assess for pulsus paradoxus when evaluating a patient for suspected cardiac tamponade.

4. List the common causes of pericarditis.

• Idiopathy
• Viral/bacterial/fungal infections
• Tuberculosis
• Post myocardial infarction/post cardiotomy syndrome (Dressler's syndrome)
• Uremia
• Neoplasm

- Radiation
- Trauma
- Autoimmune/inflammatory disease (for example, systemic lupus erythematosus, sarcoidosis, amyloidosis, rheumatoid arthritis, scleroderma)
- Drug-induced
- Dissected aortic aneurysm
- Myxedema

5. **Describe the clinical presentation that may be seen in a patient with pericarditis.**

Patients typically will complain of retrosternal chest discomfort, which is aggravated by deep breathing and lying supine and is relieved by sitting up or leaning forward. Dyspnea, fever, and leukocytosis may also be present.

Physical examination will often reveal a pericardial friction rub.

Diagnostic testing will typically demonstrate:
- ECG: generalized ST- and T-wave changes, with the initial ECG showing diffuse ST elevation followed later by a return to baseline and then T-wave inversion
- Chest radiograph: cardiac enlargement if pericardial fluid has started to accumulate
- Echocardiogram: often normal in inflammatory pericarditis but may show a pericardial effusion

6. **What is Dressler's syndrome?**

Dressler's syndrome is an illness that can be seen weeks to months after myocardial infarction or cardiac surgery. It is characterized by fever, malaise, pericarditis, leukocytosis, and pleuritic pain. Pericardial effusions and pleural effusions may be seen on radiographic and echocardiogram examinations.

7. **How much fluid does the pericardial space normally hold and how much fluid must accumulate before tamponade occurs?**

The pericardial sac normally contains 20 to 50 ml of fluid. The quantity of fluid in the pericardium when tamponade develops is variable. If fluid accumulation occurs rapidly, as little as 100 ml of fluid can cause hemodynamic compromise and tamponade. When fluid builds up slowly, 1 to 2 liters (L) of fluid can collect in the pericardial space with minimal hemodynamic effect. Thus, it is the rate of fluid accumulation in the pericardial space, not the volume, that is the most important determinant of when tamponade develops.

8. **List the common causes of constrictive pericarditis.**

- Acute pericarditis
- Tuberculosis pericarditis
- Mediastinal radiation

- Rheumatic diseases
- Sarcoidosis
- Trauma (hemopericardium)
- Cardiac surgery

9. What test is required to make a definitive diagnosis of constrictive pericarditis?

Cardiac catheterization is used to provide a definitive diagnosis of constrictive pericarditis. This test yields the hallmark sign of chronic constrictive pericarditis, which is equalization of the end-diastolic pressure to the right and left atrial and pulmonary artery pressures. If these readings are equivalent, a saline fluid challenge should be used to ascertain if occult constrictive pericarditis is present.

10. What is the incidence of primary cardiac tumors? Are primary cardiac tumors usually benign or malignant?

Primary cardiac tumors are uncommon; approximately 75% of these tumors are benign and the remaining 25% are malignant.

11. Name some benign cardiac tumors.

- Myxoma
- Lipoma
- Papillary fibroelastoma
- Rhabdomyoma
- Fibroma
- Hemangioma

12. Name the most common primary benign and primary malignant cardiac tumors in adults.

- The most common primary benign cardiac tumor is a myxoma.
- The most common primary malignant tumor is a sarcoma.

13. What percentage of benign tumors are myxomas?

Myxomas comprise 50% of all benign cardiac tumors in adults.
    While myxomas can develop in any chamber of the heart, they show a predilection for the left atrium, where 75% of all myxomas develop.

14. What symptoms would a patient with a myxoma exhibit?

While patients may present with a variety of symptoms, some of the most common include dyspnea, congestive heart failure, and syncope/presyncope. These symptoms occur as a result of the tumor interfering with normal valvular function, effectively causing valvular regurgitation or obstruction. Systemic embolizations are also commonly seen as pieces of the tumor break off and migrate. Other symptoms that patients may display are fever, lethargy, weight loss, arthralgias/myalgias, erythematous rash, and cardiac arrhythmias. On physical exam a tumor plop may be auscultated.

15. **Is surgery necessary for a patient diagnosed with a myxoma? If so, when should surgery be performed?**

An early surgical approach is indicated in the management of patients with myxomas. Many clinicians recommend performing the surgery immediately because 8% to 10% of patients die while awaiting surgery due to embolic complications.

16. **What are some common characteristics suggestive of malignant cardiac tumors?**

- Presence of distant metastasis
- Rapid growth of tumor
- Local mediastinal invasion
- Hemorrhagic pericardial effusion
- Precordial pain
- Tumor location on the right side of the heart or atrial free wall
- Combined intramural and intracavity location of tumor
- Extension into the pulmonary veins

17. **What treatment is indicated for a patient with a malignant cardiac tumor such as an angiosarcoma?**

Treatment plans vary according to the extent of metastases and primary tumor invasion. By the time most patients are diagnosed, tumor invasion and distant metastases have usually occurred, thus making treatment a palliative effort. In select patients with localized tumor growth, serial surgeries and more recently autotransplantion have been used with some success.

 Key Points

- The pericardium is comprised of visceral and parietal layers.
- Cardiac tamponade may be demonstrated by muffled heart tones, distended neck veins, hypotension, and pulsus paradoxus.
- Diffuse ST elevation on the electrocardiogram may be indicative of pericarditis.

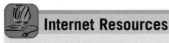

Internet Resources

American Heart Association: Circulation: Pericardial Disease:
http://circ.ahajournals.org/cgi/collection/pericardial_disease

About: Heart Disease/Cardiology:
http://heartdisease.about.com/cs/pericarditis

Bibliography

Alpert JS: *The AHA Clinical Cardiac Consult*, Philadelphia, 2001, Lippincott Williams & Wilkins.

Braunwald E: *Heart Disease: A Textbook of Cardiovascular Medicine*, ed 5, Philadelphia, 1997, WB Saunders.

Edmunds L: *Cardiac Surgery in the Adult*, New York, 1997, McGraw-Hill.

Goldman L, Braunwald E: *Primary Cardiology*, Philadelphia, 1988, WB Saunders.

Congenital Heart Disease

Kristan Devine

1. List the causes of left to right shunts.

   - Atrial septal defect (ASD)
   - Ventricular septal defect (VSD)
   - Patent ductus arteriosus (PDA)

2. What are the physiological manifestations of a left to right shunt?

   A left to right shunt causes increased blood flow through the pulmonary vascular bed that may result in congestive heart failure and pulmonary hypertension.

3. List and describe the three major types of atrial septal defects (ASD).

   Ostium primum defect: occurs in the lower portion of the atrial septum and is frequently accompanied by abnormalities in the mitral and/or tricuspid valve(s); primum defects rarely close on their own and surgery is almost always required

   Ostium secundum defect: occurs in the middle of the atrial septum

   Sinus venosous defect: usually occurs superior and posterior to the superior vena cava and is often accompanied with anomalous drainage of one or more of the pulmonary veins

4. What are some of the clinical findings associated with an ASD?

   - Systolic ejection murmur
   - Fixed splitting of the second heart sound
   - Electrocardiogram findings: incomplete right bundle branch block
   - Right ventricular hypertrophy

5. What are potential complications of an unclosed ASD?

   - Right ventricular dilatation
   - Right ventricular failure

- Pulmonary infections
- Pulmonary hypertension
- Paradoxical embolization
- Pulmonary embolus
- Arrhythmias
- Infective endocarditis

6. **When is closure of an ASD indicated?**

Surgical closure of an ASD is indicated when large left to right shunts are present with a pulmonary blood flow (Q_P) to systemic blood flow (Q_S) ratio of 1.8:1 or higher and right ventricular enlargement.

7. **What is the nonsurgical option for correcting an ASD?**

Percutaneous closure of an ASD is possible in a select group of patients. These patients have defects of the ostium secundum type and have adequate amounts of tissue in which to anchor the closing device.

8. **List the four major types of ventricular septal defect (VSD).**

- Perimembranous VSD
- Subarterial VSD
- AV canal or endocardial cushion type of VSD
- Muscular VSD

9. **What are some of the clinical features associated with ventricular septal defects?**

- Harsh and loud holosystolic murmur
- Left atrial dilatation
- Left ventricular enlargement
- Pulmonary artery dilatation

10. **When is surgical closure of a VSD indicated?**

Surgical closure of a VSD is indicated when the Q_P/Q_S ratio is greater than 1.5:1 and the calculated pulmonary vascular resistance is less than 6 units/m^2.

11. **Describe the medical management for a patient with a VSD.**

Medical management consists of afterload reduction, diuresis, and the use of cardiotonics to increase the heart's pumping efficiency.

12. **What are potential complications of an uncorrected VSD?**

- RV weakening and dilation
- Pulmonary congestion

- Pulmonary infections
- Pulmonary hypertension
- Formation of blood clots
- Arrhythmias
- Stroke

13. **What is patent ductus arteriosus (PDA)?**

PDA is the persistence of a normal fetal structure between the left pulmonary artery and the descending aorta. It usually closes within 24 hours after birth, but in some infants it may remain patent. Persistence beyond 10 days of life is considered abnormal.

14. **What are the physiological effects of a patent ductus arteriosus (PDA)?**

The effect is usually dependent on the degree of the left to right shunt and the ability of the heart to handle the increased volume. A large PDA may lead to increased pulmonary vascular resistance.

15. **What are the clinical manifestations of a PDA?**
- May be asymptomatic
- Loud machinery murmur
- Hyperactive precordium
- Widened pulse pressure
- Bounding pulse
- Congestive heart failure
- Cardiomegaly

16. **What are the treatment options for PDA?**
- Surgical closure
- Catheter closure

17. **What are the potential complications associated with an uncorrected PDA?**
- Congestive heart failure
- Bacterial endocarditis
- Aneurysm of the ductus
- Pulmonary hypertension

18. **Why are scuba divers with a patent foramen ovale (PFO) more likely to suffer a stroke?**

Decompression gas bubbles normally travel through the veins, but in an individual with a PFO these bubbles may travel through the PFO from the right side of the heart to the left side of the heart. The gas bubbles can then be pumped into the systemic circulation, possibly resulting in a stroke.

19. What is tetralogy of Fallot (TOF)?

Tetralogy of Fallot is a congenital cardiac condition characterized by four specific defects (hence its name):
- Pulmonary valve stenosis or atresia
- Ventricular septal defect
- Overriding aorta
- Right ventricular hypertrophy

20. What are the primary clinical findings in patients with TOF?

- Cyanosis
- Hypoxia
- Loud systolic murmur

21. What therapeutic options may be used in treating patients with TOF?

- Oxygen therapy
- Phlebotomy if the hematocrit is greater than 65%
- Exchange transfusions
- Pulmonic valve balloon dilatation

22. How is the tetralogy of Fallot surgically repaired?

Surgical repair of the tetralogy of Fallot consists of widening the pulmonic valve (repair/replacement) and closure of the VSD. Surgical correction of the aorta is not required.

23. What is coarctation of the aorta?

Coarctation of the aorta is a malformation in which the walls of the aorta are narrowed or pinched. While this narrowing can occur anywhere along the aorta, it typically occurs just beyond the subclavian artery.

24. What is the physiological hallmark of coarctation of the aorta?

Systemic hypertension

25. What are the common clinical manifestations in patients with coarctation of the aorta?

- Delayed or absent femoral pulse compared to the right brachial pulse
- Blood pressure differentials between the upper and lower extremities (systolic blood pressure [SBP] for upper extremity greater than SBP for lower extremity)
- Widened pulse pressure
- Aortic ejection murmur

26. **What other congenital abnormality is frequently seen in patients with coarctation of the aorta?**

A bicuspid aortic valve can be found in up to 80% of patients with coarctation of the aorta.

27. **What is Marfan syndrome?**

It is a connective tissue disorder that affects the skeletal, cardiovascular, and ocular systems.

28. **What are the physical stigmata usually associated with Marfan syndrome?**
- Displacement of the ocular lens
- Arachnodactyly
- Tall, lanky extremities
- Chest wall deformities
- High riding arched palate
- Hyperextensibility of the joints
- Sparse muscle mass
- Scoliosis

29. **When caring for a 30-year-old patient with Marfan syndrome, what abnormalities can one expect to see on an echocardiogram?**

Patients with Marfan syndrome will typically have aortic root dilatation and mitral valve prolapse with mitral regurgitation. The aortic root dilation is progressive in nature and may be complicated by aortic insufficiency, aortic dissection, and rupture.

30. **What is the gold standard for diagnosing anomalies of the coronary arteries?**

The gold standard for diagnosing coronary abnormalities is cardiac catheterization and angiocardiography.

31. **What abnormalities of the coronary arteries may occur?**

Coronary abnormalities may include abnormal anatomy, abnormal coronary course, and anomalies intrinsic to the coronary artery such as coronary artery aneurysm or myocardial bridging.

32. **Why is a patient at high risk for sudden death when their coronary artery extends between the aorta and pulmonary artery?**

This patient is at risk for sudden death because of ischemia caused by the slitlike ostium of the coronary artery and compression of the coronary between the aortic and pulmonic roots.

33. **What are some of the maternal conditions that may contribute to the development of congenital heart disease?**
    - Rubella infection
    - Cytomegalovirus infection
    - Poor nutrition
    - Coxsackie infection
    - Family history of cardiac disease

34. **List innocent murmurs noted in childhood.**
    - Precordial vibratory murmur (Still's murmur)
    - Pulmonary ejection systolic murmur
    - Supraclavicular arterial bruit

35. **Describe the characteristics associated with innocent murmurs.**

Murmur	Characteristics
Precordial vibratory murmur	Soft midsystolic murmur, heard at left lower sternal border; softens or disappears with standing and is accentuated with squatting
Pulmonary ejection systolic murmur	Early systolic ejection murmur; heard at left parasternal border and may radiate to left neck; most commonly heard in adolescents
Subclavian arterial bruit	Harsh, crescendo-decrescendo systolic ejection murmur loudest at right supraclavicular area; compression of subclavian area may diminish sound

36. **Describe features of functional murmurs.**
    - Usually do not radiate
    - Disappear with inspiratory effort
    - Vary with patient position
    - Are less than grade 3

Key Points

- Left to right shunts are caused by VSD, ASD, and PDA.
- Complications of an uncorrected VSD include right ventricle failure, pulmonary hypertension, stroke, arrhythmias, and thromboembolic events.
- Marfan syndrome is a connective tissue disorder that affects the cardiovascular, musculoskeletal, and ocular systems.

Internet Resources

MH Online: Medical Humanities: Congenital Heart Disease:
http://www.medhums.com/cgi/collection/congenital_heart_disease

Heart Center Online: For Cardiologists and Their Patients:
http://www.heartcenteronline.com

Bibliography

Alpert JS: *The AHA Clinical Cardiac Consult*, Philadelphia, 2001, Lippincott Williams & Wilkins.

Braunwald E: *Heart Disease: A Textbook of Cardiovascular Medicine*, ed 5, Philadelphia, 1997, WB Saunders.

Edmunds L: *Cardiac Surgery in the Adult*, New York, 1997, McGraw-Hill.

Heartcenteronline: www.heartcenteronline.com, 2003.

Preoperative Evaluation

Sandra Davis

1. What is the purpose of the preoperative evaluation?

A preoperative (pre-op) evaluation is performed to assess and predict both the perioperative (peri-op) and the postoperative (post-op) morbidity and mortality risk of a patient. A comprehensive and systematic assessment of the patient before cardiac surgery is crucial because peri-op and post-op complications can be minimized by a well-planned pre-op evaluation.

2. What major complications of cardiac surgery are associated with increased morbidity and should be preoperatively assessed?

Complications can occur in any body system following cardiac surgery. It is particularly important for the nurse to preoperatively identify those patients who may be at risk for neurological abnormalities, wound infections, and renal dysfunction.

3. What are the predictors of mortality for the patient undergoing coronary artery bypass graft (CABG) surgery?

According to the American College of Cardiology/American Heart Association (ACC/AHA) guidelines for CABG surgery, there are seven variables that are predictive of mortality after CABG surgery:
- Urgency of operation
- Age
- Prior heart surgery
- Gender
- Left ventricular ejection fraction (LVEF)
- Percent stenosis of the left main coronary artery
- Number of major arteries with >70% stenosis

4. What is the mortality risk for a patient undergoing CABG surgery?

For patients having elective CABG surgery who are less than 65 years of age and who do not have a severely depressed LVEF or congestive heart failure (CHF), the 30-day mortality risk is <1%. For patients less than 65 years of age who have an LVEF of 25% to 35% and no other comorbidities, first-time CABG has an operative risk of <5%.

5. **How is the pre-op evaluation for off-pump coronary artery bypass (OPCAB) patients different than that for patients having traditional CABG surgery with cardiopulmonary bypass (CPB)?**

Many surgeons follow the same preparations for the OPCAB patient as for the CABG with CPB patient. This is done in anticipation of an emergency or any other situation that may arise during surgery that necessitates placing the patient on CPB. While OPCAB patients still undergo a median sternotomy and graft harvesting, CPB is eliminated, and grafts are anastamosed to target vessels while the heart is still beating. Stabilizing devices are utilized for the heart.

6. **What are the advantages of OPCAB surgery?**

It is believed that OPCAB surgery may reduce complications and improve outcome in high-risk patients. High-risk patients generally: (a) are older than 70 years of age, (b) have carotid disease or are at risk for stroke, (c) have kidney disease, and/or (d) have lung disease. A recent study has shown that OPCAB surgery offers substantial benefits for diabetic patients. It is also believed that OPCAB patients require fewer blood transfusions, are extubated sooner, and are released earlier from the hospital. There is a growing trend toward OPCAB utilization in all patients undergoing CABG surgery.

7. **What is the most important criterion used to assess a patient's risk for post-op complication?**

A detailed history with documentation of significant findings is probably the most important criterion in assessing the patient's risk of having a post-op complication.

8. **What aspects of the patient's history should be the focus of attention for the preoperative nurse?**

The nurse should focus on several areas. It is extremely important that the nurse not only inquires about diseases and procedures but also asks questions in a manner that the patient understands. The major areas of focus when obtaining a patient history are listed below.

History of present illness:
- Type of heart disease and associated symptoms
- Associated symptoms
- Chest pain, discomfort with or without radiation
- Palpitations
- Shortness of breath
- Dyspnea on exertion
- Paroxysmal nocturnal dyspnea

- Fatigue
- Syncope or presyncope
- Lower extremity edema
- Cough
- Gastrointestinal (GI) symptoms
- Diaphoresis
- Nausea/vomiting

History of prior cardiac disease:
- CAD
- Angina
- Aortic aneurysm
- Myocardial infarction (MI)
- Congestive heart failure (CHF)
- Pulmonary edema
- Arrhythmias
- Valvular heart disease
- Endocarditis
- Congenital heart disease
- Rheumatic fever

Risk factors for CAD:
- Diabetes mellitus
- Hypertension
- Dyslipidemia
- Cigarette smoking
- Obesity
- Sedentary life-style
- Family history
- Age
- Race

Conditions associated with CAD:
- Peripheral vascular disease
- Cerebrovascular disease
- Renal insufficiency

Presence of coexisting diseases such as:
- Respiratory diseases
- GI disturbances

Past medical history:
- Gastric and peptic ulcers
- Anemia
- Blood transfusions
- Corticosteroid use
- Radiation to chest
- Risk for coagulopathy

Past surgical history

Occupational and social history:
- Alcohol use
- Tobacco use
- Illicit drug use

Medications (dose and frequency):
- Prescription
- Over the counter
- Home remedies
- Herbals

Allergies and reactions
Functional capacity
Social and family support systems
Emotional readiness for the operation
Understanding of the illness/impact of the illness

9. **What are the components of the physical examination?**

Vital signs:
- Height, weight, temperature, blood pressure in both extremities, pulse, respiratory rate
- Body mass index (BMI)

HEENT exam:
- Cranial nerves
- Jugular venous distention
- Carotid bruits

Cardiac exam:
- Heart rate and rhythm
- Point of maximum impulse
- Heart sounds
- Murmurs, clicks, rubs, gallops

Chest exam:
- Respiratory rate
- Breath sounds
- Adventitious sounds

Abdominal exam:
- Bowel sounds
- Renal or abdominal bruits
- Liver span

Extremity exam:
- Peripheral edema
- Peripheral pulses, color, and temperature
- Evidence of previous vein surgery
- Muscle strength
- Sensation

10. **What baseline diagnostic tests are required for the patient undergoing cardiac surgery?**

- Complete blood count with differential
- Comprehensive metabolic panel
- Prothrombin time
- Partial thromboplastin time

- Bleeding time
- Urinalysis
- Chest x-ray
- Electrocardiogram (ECG)

11. What invasive and noninvasive diagnostic tests and procedures are usually obtained as part of a patient work-up before cardiac surgery?

- Transthoracic echocardiography
- Transesophageal echocardiography
- Stress or exercise echocardiography
- Exercise stress testing
- Pharmacologic stress testing
- Cardiac catheterization

12. What is an echocardiogram (Echo)?

This diagnostic test uses beams of ultrasonic waves to record the position and motion of the heart and its internal structures. Transducers can be applied directly to the skin on the chest (transthoracic Echo) or a transducer can be introduced into the esophagus (transesophageal Echo) to provide two-dimensional images of the heart. Echocardiogram tests are usually required for patients with valvular heart disease or cardiomyopathy. An Echo not only assesses the size and structure of the heart and its chambers but also measures heart and heart valve functioning. It can determine the LVEF, wall motion abnormalities, valvular abnormalities, tumors, thrombi, and septal defects.

13. Describe stress echocardiography.

This procedure enhances the sensitivity and specificity of detecting CAD by recording echocardiograms during rest, exercise (stress), and recovery to show the functional capacity of the patient's heart. Patients may exercise on a treadmill, or the heart may be stressed by pharmacologic means with medications such as dobutamine.

14. Describe exercise stress testing.

This test yields valuable information about a patient's ischemic threshold and functional capacity as it determines how well the heart works during physical activity. An ECG is recorded before exercise, at peak exercise, and after exercise to determine the heart's functional capacity. The specificity of a stress test may be improved with the injection of thallium (a radioactive tracer; Cardiolite is another radioactive tracer) during exercise. If a patient has ischemia, the involved area of the myocardium does not initially absorb the thallium, and a defect appears on a myocardial perfusion scan. As the patient recovers from exercise, the ischemia is displayed and the defect fills. It may also show conduction abnormalities and/or arrhythmias.

15. **Describe the pharmacologic stress test.**

This is also called chemical stress imaging. This type of nuclear stress testing uses adenosine, dobutamine, or Persantine to stimulate the heart in patients who are not able to exercise (for example, those with arthritis, pulmonary disease, or peripheral vascular disease).

16. **What is the role of cardiac catherization in evaluating patients for cardiac surgery?**

Most patients undergoing cardiac surgery will have a cardiac catheterization before surgery. This procedure helps visualize the coronary anatomy and the location of coronary blockages. It is the only definitive means for identifying CAD and is indicated for patients with CAD or valvular heart disease. A right heart catheterization provides information about the filling pressures of the heart, the pulmonary artery pressures, cardiac output, oxygen saturation, and tricuspid and pulmonic valve functioning. Radiopaque dye may be used to visualize the left side of the heart (angiogram). The left heart catheterization provides information about pressures in the aortic root, the left atrium, and the left ventricle, the LVEF, and mitral and aortic valve functioning. An arteriogram gives information about coronary anatomy.

A ventriculogram may also be conducted to determine left ventricular function and any mitral valve abnormalities. An aortogram would show any abnormalities of the aorta and aortic valve.

17. **What additional diagnostic studies may be required for the patient undergoing cardiac surgery?**

- Carotid ultrasound may be required if the patient has audible carotid bruits or has a history of carotid artery disease, cerebral vascular accident, or transient ischemic attack. A carotid ultrasound should be obtained for a patient who has a cardiac murmur that radiates into the carotid arteries.
- Lower extremity ultrasound: Doppler, duplex, and color flow Doppler ultrasounds may be required if the patient has a history of intermittent claudication or arterial insufficiency. It may also be used to rule out deep vein thrombosis in a patient with a history or physical exam suggestive of the diagnosis.
- Vein mapping may be required by some surgeons to determine the caliber and quality of veins before they are harvested.
- Arterial blood gas may need to be obtained in patients with respiratory disease.
- Pulmonary function tests may be required pre-op for those patients with severe pulmonary disease.
- Dental evaluation and clearance are required for all patients who are undergoing valvular heart surgery. Dental infection is a source of bacterial endocarditis; therefore all infected teeth must be pulled and abscesses must be drained before surgery. Dentists may also require panoramic dental radiographs as part of the evaluation before surgery.

18. **What are the indications for an intraaortic balloon pump (IABP) before cardiac surgery?**

An intraaortic balloon pump may be used preoperatively for stabilization of the high-risk patient. It is crucial to identify those patients who may need close monitoring and intervention during the pre-op period. Patients with accelerating angina or who develop angina at rest are high-risk patients. Patients with acute myocardial ischemia may develop cardiogenic shock with ventricular arrhythmias or pulmonary edema. In addition to the IABP, these patients may require pre-op intubation, mechanical ventilation, and urgent revascularization. Patients who have been diagnosed with left main coronary artery disease are usually supported with the balloon pump before surgery.

19. **Are there special preparations for the same-day-admission cardiac surgery patient?**

More and more low-risk elective cardiac surgery patients are being admitted on the day of their operation. In this case the nurse has not had the opportunity to monitor the patient overnight. In addition the patient may not have been in contact with a health care provider for days to weeks. Therefore it is important for the nurse to ask specifically about recent respiratory tract infections, fever, chills, and signs and symptoms of a urinary tract infection. Patients should not have had anything to eat or drink after midnight the night before surgery. The nurse should also determine when the patient consumed their last alcoholic drink.

Institutions vary on the length of time for which preoperative laboratory data are acceptable. If the patient has had a recent cardiac catheterization, electrolytes and creatinine must be obtained to ensure adequate renal functioning after the dye-load.

The nurse should also answer any questions that the patient may have concerning their operation and hospital stay as well as alleviate any anxieties of the patient or the patient's family members.

20. **What medications are stopped before cardiac surgery?**

Warfarin (Coumadin) is generally discontinued 5 to 7 days before surgery. Depending on the condition for which the Coumadin was prescribed, it may be necessary to initiate heparin upon discontinuation of the Coumadin. Nonsteroidal antiinflammatory drugs (NSAIDs) and cyclooxygenase-2 (COX-2) inhibitors are usually discontinued 5 to 7 days before surgery. It is not necessary to stop aspirin before surgery; the cardiologist and surgeon will make that decision. Plavix is usually withheld at least 48 hours before cardiac surgery. Diuretics and oral hypoglycemics are withheld the day of surgery. One third to one half of the NPH insulin dose is given the morning of surgery. Generally, medications used to control angina, blood pressure, or arrhythmias are not discontinued.

21. What types of patients are at risk for bleeding during cardiac surgery?

Any patient undergoing cardiac surgery may need blood during or after the operation. Patients who are having repeated operations, patients who are undergoing combined procedures, elderly or debilitated patients, patients with pre-op anemia, patients requiring ventricular aneurysmectomy or endocardial resection, and patients with abnormal bleeding studies are at a greater risk for bleeding.

22. Is blood ordered for all patients undergoing cardiac surgery?

Usually patients are typed and screened for blood; then blood products are held in reserve for potential use. Other blood components that may be used are fresh frozen plasma and platelets. Because of the limited supply and the risk of infection, homologous blood donations are used with discretion.

23. Many patients request autologous blood donations before cardiac surgery. What are the contraindications?

If the surgery is scheduled several weeks in advance and if the patient's medical condition permits, autologous donations may be arranged. However, patients must recover from any anemia after the donation before surgery is permitted. Iron or erythropoietin may be given to aid in this process. Family and friends with compatible blood types may donate blood. Depending on the institution and the Red Cross organization in your area, several days are needed for directed donor blood donations.

24. What preparation is required the night before cardiac surgery?

Patients must not eat or drink anything after midnight the night before surgery. Patients are also required to shower with an antibacterial soap to reduce the potential for wound infection. Any shaving of the skin that is required is usually done in the operating room before the start of the operation. A pre-op enema is not required. A sleeping medication may help alleviate anxiety but should be used with caution in elderly, frail, confused, or demented patients. Sedation should not be given the day of the procedure unless the consent form has been signed and a sedative has been ordered. Unstable patients should not be sedated until they are in the operating room.

25. What items are included in a preoperative checklist?

- Name of the planned procedure
- Laboratory test results
- Diagnostic studies
- Chest x-ray report
- Surgical team's pre-op note
- Anesthesia's pre-op note
- Type, screen, and cross-match blood on hold in blood bank
- Antibiotic orders

- Antiseptic scrub/shower completed
- NPO after midnight
- Pre-op medications per anesthesia
- Signed consent form

 Key Points

- A preoperative (pre-op) evaluation is performed to assess and predict both the perioperative (peri-op) and the postoperative (post-op) morbidity and mortality risk of a patient.
- Factors that may affect outcome after coronary bypass surgery include: age, urgency of surgery, prior heart surgery, gender, left ventricular function, and number of coronaries grafted.
- Preoperative teaching is an important aspect of preparation for the patient undergoing cardiac surgery.

 Internet Resources

Cardio Thoracic Surgery Notes:
http://www.ctsnet.org/residents/ctsn

American College of Surgeons: College Guidelines:
http://www.facs.org/fellows_info/guidelines/cardiac.html

Bibliography

Cohn SL, Goldman L: Preoperative risk evaluation and perioperative management of patients with coronary artery disease, *Med Clin N Am* 87(1):111-136, 2003.

Eagle RA, Guyton RA, Ewy GA, Fonges J, Gardner TJ et al: American College of Cardiology/American Heart Association: *Guidelines for Coronary Artery Bypass Graft Surgery*: A Report of the American College of Cardiology/American Heart Association Task Force on Practice Guidelines, *Journal of the American College of Cardiology*, 34:1262-346, 1999.

Finkelmeier BA: *Cardiothoracic surgical nursing*, ed 2, Philadelphia, 2000, Lippincott.

Way LW, Doherty GM: *Current surgical diagnosis and treatment*, ed 11, New York, 2003, McGraw-Hill.

Hemodynamic Monitoring and Vasoactive Medications

Kristan Devine

1. **Briefly describe the three stages of shock.**

   Compensatory stage: Compensatory mechanisms cause vasoconstriction, thereby maintaining normal blood pressure and adequate perfusion to vital organs.

   Decompensated or progressive stage: Patient's compensatory mechanisms are no longer able to maintain adequate perfusion to vital organs and signs and symptoms of circulatory and metabolic imbalances are seen. End-organ injury is reversible at this stage.

   Irreversible or refractory stage: Irreversible cellular damage has occurred because of prolonged hypoperfusion with resultant permanent tissue and end-organ damage.

2. **Describe the hemodynamic profile in a patient with cardiogenic shock.**

   - Normal or decreased blood pressure
   - Increased pulmonary artery pressure
   - Increased pulmonary arterial wedge pressure (PAWP) and left ventricular end-diastolic pressure (LVEDP)
   - Normal or increased central venous pressure (CVP)
   - Increased systemic vascular resistance (SVR)
   - Decreased cardiac output (CO)/cardiac index (CI)
   - Decreased mixed venous oxygen saturation (SVO_2)

3. **List the differential diagnoses for a patient in cardiogenic shock.**

   - Myocardial infarction (MI)
   - Cardiomyopathy
   - Pericardial tamponade
   - Massive pulmonary embolus
   - Tension pneumothorax
   - Tachyarrhythmias or bradyarrhythmias
   - Valvular obstruction
   - Acute myocarditis
   - Pressure on inferior vena cava (pregnant women)

4. **What direct and indirect information is obtained from hemodynamic monitoring?**
   - Blood volume
   - Cardiac pump effectiveness
   - Tissue perfusion
   - Vascular capacitance

5. **What potential complications can be associated with pulmonary artery catheter placement?**
   - Infection
   - Pneumothorax
   - Hematoma at the insertion site
   - Right ventricular perforation
   - Arrhythmias
   - Pulmonary artery rupture

6. **In what order should hemodynamic parameters be addressed?**
   - Heart rate (HR) and rhythm
   - Preload
   - Afterload
   - Contractility

7. **Which hemodynamic factors reflect preload?**
   - Right atrial pressure (CVP)
   - Pulmonary artery wedge pressure
   - Right ventricular end-diastolic volume

8. **Which hemodynamic factors reflect afterload?**
   - Pulmonary vascular resistance
   - Systemic vascular resistance

9. **List the normal ranges for hemodynamic and physiologic measurements in the adult patient.**
   - Pulmonary artery pressure (PAP): 15 to 25/8 to 15 mm Hg
   - Right atrial pressure (CVP): 2 to 6 mm Hg
   - Pulmonary artery wedge pressure (PAWP): 4 to 12 mm Hg
   - Cardiac output (CO): 4 to 8 L/min
   - Cardiac index (CI): 2.5 to 4.2 L/min/m^2
   - Systemic vascular resistance (SVR): 660 to 1500 dynes/sec/cm^{-5}
   - Pulmonary vascular resistance (PVR): 20 to 120 dynes/sec/cm^{-5}
   - Arterial blood pressure (ABP): 100 to 130/60 to 90 mm Hg (mean 70 to 105 mm Hg)
   - Left ventricular end-diastolic pressure (LVEDP): 4 to 12 mm Hg
   - Left ventricular systolic pressure: 100 to 130 mm Hg

10. **What four factors determine cardiac output?**

Cardiac output (CO) is the product of heart rate and stroke volume (SV):

$$CO = HR \times SV$$

Stroke volume is the amount of blood that is ejected from the heart with each contraction and is influenced by: (1) preload, (2) afterload, and (3) contractility.

Thus the four factors that affect an individual's cardiac output (CO) are:

- Heart rate
- Preload
- Afterload
- Contractility

11. **What quick assessment can be used to determine adequate cardiac output?**

The presence of pedal pulses indicates a minimal cardiac index of 2.0 L, the level necessary to maintain perfusion of the microcirculation.

12. **Describe the hemodynamic profile of a patient with severe aortic stenosis.**

- Decreased pulse pressure
- Normal or increased SVR
- Normal PVR
- Normal ABP
- Normal or increased PAP
- Normal or increased PAWP
- Normal or decreased CO
- Normal or decreased SVO_2

13. **Describe the hemodynamic and physiologic effects of an intraaortic balloon pump (IABP).**

Balloon inflation at the onset of diastole:
- Increases coronary and cerebral perfusion
- Increases systemic perfusion

Balloon deflation during systole:
- Decreases afterload, myocardial workload, and oxygen consumption
- Increases stroke volume and cardiac output
- Decreases LV preload (PWP)

14. **Are thermodilution cardiac output measurements accurate in a patient with severe tricuspid regurgitation (TR)?**

Thermodilution cardiac output measurements are NOT accurate in a patient with severe TR because both the patient's blood and the cold injectate recirculate in the right heart chambers as a result of the backward flow of blood from the right ventricle into the right atrium.

15. **What is the significance of "v" waves?**

   In the ECG "v" waves can be seen in CVP and PCW tracings just after the T wave; "v" waves are a result of the atrium filling with blood before the opening of the mitral and tricuspid valves.

   Large "v" waves seen in pulmonary artery waveforms are indicative of mitral regurgitation.

   Large "v" waves seen in central venous waveforms are indicative of tricuspid regurgitation.

16. **A patient in the intensive care unit has severe mitral stenosis (MS). His hemodynamic parameters show a PAWP of 12 mm Hg. Is this patient hypovolemic, normovolemic, or hypervolemic? Explain your answer.**

   The patient is hypovolemic. Patients with severe mitral stenosis (MS) are volume-dependent and may require a PAWP of approximately 35 mm Hg to maintain adequate ventricle filling and cardiac index.

17. **In evaluating a patient with a new aortic insufficiency (AI) murmur, a grade 2/6 diastolic murmur at the left sternal border is heard. His blood pressure is 160/30 mm Hg. Does this patient have chronic or acute AI?**

   The patient has chronic AI as evidenced by his widened pulse pressure. Systolic blood pressure is elevated in chronic AI as a result of the increased regurgitant stroke volume entering the aorta and systemic circulation. Diastolic blood pressure, however, is decreased due to compensatory vasodilatation and reflux of aortic blood into the left ventricle.

18. **List three factors that can adversely affect SVO$_2$.**

   - Increased metabolic demands (for example, shivering)
   - Poor oxygenation
   - Decreased cardiac output

19. **Describe the clinical presentation of low cardiac output states (LCOS).**

   - Cool, clammy skin
   - Poor capillary refill
   - Oliguria
   - Restlessness/agitation
   - Tachypnea
   - Metabolic acidosis

20. **List the differential diagnoses for LCOS.**

   - Myocardial ischemia
   - Myocardial dysfunction/pump failure
   - Hypovolemia
   - Tamponade
   - Hypothermia

21. **How do you calculate systemic vascular resistance (SVR)?**

$$SVR = [(MAP - CVP)/CO] \times 80$$

22. **How are cardiac output (CO) and cardiac index (CI) calculated? Which measurement is more valuable in evaluating a patient's condition?**

$$CO = SV \times HR$$
$$CI = CO/BSA$$

CI is more valuable because it takes into account the patient's body size (BSA = body surface area).

23. **Name the four receptor sites where vasoactive medications work and describe their actions at each site.**
    - **Alpha-adrenergic receptors:** vasoconstriction
    - **Beta receptors:** increase atrial and ventricular contraction, increase heart rate by stimulating the SA node and enhancing AV conduction
    - **Beta$_2$ receptors:** bronchodilation and vasodilatation
    - **Dopaminergic receptors:** vasodilatation in coronary, renal, mesenteric, and cerebrovascular beds

24. **Why are arterial vasodilators used cautiously in patients with severe aortic stenosis?**

Patients with severe aortic stenosis have a relatively fixed stroke volume and therefore rely on vasoconstriction to maintain adequate blood pressure and cardiac output.

25. **You are caring for a patient with SAM (systolic anterior motion of the mitral valve leaflet). What drugs are contraindicated in this patient and why?**

The use of beta-adrenergic agonists and digitalis would be contraindicated because they would increase the gradient across the left ventricular outflow tract. While not contraindicated, diuretics must be used cautiously in these patients.

26. **How do you treat a patient who has developed hypotension related to a calcium channel blocker?**

Administer calcium and increase fluid volume.

27. What are the indications for beta-blocker therapy?

- Acute myocardial infarction
- Rate control of atrial arrhythmias
- Conversion to normal sinus rhythm (NSR)
- Emergency antihypertensive therapy in the presence of a stroke

28. Why are beta-blockers indicated in patients with acute and chronic coronary disease?

The early administration of beta-blockers in patients with acute MIs has been shown to limit infarct size and decrease the incidence of ventricular fibrillation and cardiac rupture. Studies have also shown that beta-blockers reduce the risk of reinfarction and death in patients undergoing both acute treatment for a myocardial infarction and long-term treatment for coronary disease.

29. What are the physiologic benefits of angiotensin-converting enzyme (ACE) inhibitors?

- Increase LV function and cardiac output
- Increase renal, coronary, and cerebral blood flow
- Decrease preload
- Decrease end-diastolic pressure
- Decrease afterload
- Are mixed arterial and venous dilators
- Cause no change in heart rate or myocardial contractility
- Cause no neurohormonal activation
- Have resultant diuresis and natriuresis

30. What are the contraindications to the use of ACE inhibitors?

- Renal artery stenosis
- Renal insufficiency (relative)
- Hyperkalemia
- Arterial hypotension
- Cough
- Angioedema
- Pregnancy (may cause fetal injury or death)

31. What are the beneficial hemodynamic effects of digoxin?

- Increased cardiac output
- Increased left ventricular ejection fraction
- Decreased left ventricular diastolic pressure
- Increased exercise tolerance
- Increased natriuresis
- Decreased neurohormonal activation

32. In what clinical conditions should digoxin be avoided?

Avoided:
- Pericardial disease
- Restrictive cardiomyopathy
- Mitral stenosis (unless atrial fibrillation is present)

Contraindicated:
- Hypertrophic cardiomyopathy
- AV conduction blocks

33. What are the primary indications for epinephrine infusion?
- Complete heart block
- Ventricular standstill
- Anaphylaxis
- Refractory asthma
- Cardiac surgery

34. How is epinephrine administered?

Epinephrine can be administered by intravenous infusion or by direct-push or intracardiac injection. The infusion concentration is usually 1 to 8 mg in 250 ml of fluid. The intracardiac or direct-push dose is usually 1 mg. Epinephrine may also be administered through an endotracheal tube, the usual dose being 0.1 to 1 mg of 1:10,000 solution.

35. What is milrinone (Primacor)?

Milrinone is a phosphodiesterase inhibitor. It improves the contractility of the myocardium, increases cardiac output (CO), and decreases ventricular filling and PCW pressures. There is little or no change seen in heart rate or blood pressure.

36. What is Natrecor (nesiritide)?

Natrecor is a recombinant form of human B-type natriuretic peptide, a naturally occurring protein secreted by the heart as part of the body's response to acute heart failure. Natrecor is approved for the intravenous treatment of patients with acutely decompensated congestive heart failure.

37. You are caring for a patient that is being infused with sodium nitroprusside (Nipride). What is the metabolite of Nipride and what are the signs of toxicity?

Nitroprusside is metabolized to cyanide and then to thiocyanate, which is then excreted by the kidneys. Toxicity can occur with prolonged use or infusion of high doses. The signs of thiocyanate toxicity that may need to be monitored include tinnitus, blurred vision, altered mental status, nausea, abdominal pain, hyperreflexia, and seizures. The antidote is sodium thiosulfate.

38. List common intravenous pharmacologic agents used to treat cardiac surgery patients.

Common intravenous pharmacologic agents used to treat cardiac surgery patients

Agent	Indication	Dosage	Special Considerations
Nitroprusside (Nipride)	Hypertension and elevated systemic vascular resistance; dilates peripheral vessels directly	0.1-0.25 mcg/kg/min, with upward titration to 8 mcg/kg/min	Severe hypotension may develop but duration is very short; filling pressures should be optimized before initiation; usage longer than 24 hours may be associated with alteration in mental status and worsening respiratory function; adjust for patient with renal dysfunction, should not exceed 3 mcg/kg/min
Epinephrine	Stimulates alpha and beta-adrenergic receptors	1-8 mcg/min	Tachycardia; monitor blood glucose levels; may worsen acidosis
Dobutamine (Dobutrex)	Inotropic effect; stimulates $beta_1$-adrenergic receptors	2-20 mcg/kg/min	Monitor for arrhythmias
Dopamine	Hypotension and shock; stimulates alpha, $beta_1$-adrenergic, and dopaminergic receptors	2-20 mcg/kg/min	Tachycardia and arrhythmias; should administer via central line; may cause tissue necrosis if infiltrates peripherally
Nitroglycerin	Myocardial ischemia and lowered central and pulmonary filling pressures	5-200 mcg/min	Hypotension
Norepinephrine (Levophed)	Shock; stimulates alpha and $beta_1$-adrenergic receptors	2-12 mcg/min intravenous infusion; refractory shock may require up to 30 mcg/min	Hypertension, arrhythmias, and anaphylaxis; may exacerbate asthma
Milrinone (Primacor)	Inhibits cyclic AMP phosphodiesterase	Loading dosage of 50 mcg/kg over a 10-min period and then infusion from 0.375 to 0.75 mcg/kg/min	Monitor for ventricular arrhythmias; adjust for renal dysfunction

Data from Marso SP, Griffin BP, Topol EJ: *Manual of Cardiovascular Medicine*, Philadelphia, 2000, Lippincott Williams & Wilkins.

Key Points

* The three stages of shock are compensatory, decompensated, and refractory.
* Heart rate, preload, afterload, and contractility should be addressed in the hemodynamic profile of all patients.
* Vasodilator medications affect the alpha-adrenergic, beta, and dopaminergic receptors.

Internet Resources

Hemodynamics:
http://www.cvphysiology.com/Hemodynamics

University of Wisconsin Department of Anesthesiology: Hemodynamic Monitoring and Inotropes:
http://www.anesthesia.wisc.edu/med3/Hemodynamic/hemodynamic.html

Bibliography

Braunwald E: *Heart Disease: A Textbook of Cardiovascular Medicine*, ed 5, Philadelphia, 1997, WB Saunders.

Gawlinski A, Hamwi D: *Acute Care Nurse Practitioner: Clinical Curriculum and Certification Review*, Philadelphia, 1999, WB Saunders.

Hazinski MF, Cummins RO, Field JM: *Handbook of Emergency Cardiovascular Care*, Tex, 2000, American Heart Association.

Isselbacher KJ, Braunwald E, Wilson JD, Martin JB, Fauci AS, Kasper DL: *Harrison's Principles of Internal Medicine*, ed 15, New York, 2001, McGraw-Hill.

Marso SP, Griffin BP, Topol EJ: *Manual of Cardiovascular Medicine*, Philadelphia, 2000, Lippincott Williams & Wilkins.

Chapter 14

Anesthesia for Cardiac Surgery

Scott A. Schartel

1. What is the preanesthesia assessment?

The preanesthesia assessment includes:
- Focused history and physical examination
- Review of indicated diagnostic studies
- Assessment of the patient's fitness for anesthesia and the risks associated with anesthesia
- Formulation of an anesthetic plan

2. What should be the focus of the history in a patient's preanesthesia assessment?

The history seeks to gather information about medical and surgical diseases and conditions, medication and environmental allergies, and current medication therapy. In general, the history concentrates most heavily on the cardiac and pulmonary systems, because these systems have the most impact on the course of an anesthetic.

Review of the cardiac system identifies the presence of hypertension, angina, prior myocardial infarction, heart failure, valvular heart disease, and symptoms associated with these conditions. Identification of factors that precipitate symptoms is also sought.

Review of the pulmonary system identifies current or past episodes of pulmonary edema, asthma, chronic obstructive lung disease, tuberculosis, and pneumonia. Smoking history is also reviewed. Quantification of the severity of lung diseases is sought by further questioning related to the factors that exacerbate or improve respiratory symptoms.

Previous anesthetic experiences are reviewed to identify prior problems with anesthesia. It is also important to seek evidence of untoward anesthetic events in close relatives, specifically a history of malignant hyperthermia.

3. What is malignant hyperthermia?

Malignant hyperthermia is a genetic disease that can result in a severe, and potentially fatal, hypermetabolic state when affected individuals are exposed to volatile inhalation anesthetics or succinylcholine.

4. **How is exercise tolerance assessed?**

Exercise tolerance is assessed by identifying the maximum level of physical activity that a patient can perform. For example, patients can be queried about how far they can walk without stopping, how many stairs they can climb without stopping, and their ability to perform various activities of daily living, such as carrying groceries, pushing a vacuum cleaner, or pushing a lawn mower. Exercise tolerance provides a rough estimate of cardiopulmonary reserve.

5. **What are the risk factors that predispose patients to aspiration during the induction of anesthesia?**

- Gastroesophageal reflux
- Conditions associated with decreased gastric motility and emptying (diabetes mellitus with autonomic dysfunction, obesity, pregnancy)
- Conditions associated with increased gastric volume (recent food ingestion, gastric outlet obstruction)
- Esophageal dysfunction or disease

6. **What should be the focus of the physical examination in a patient's preanesthesia assessment?**

The physical examination concentrates on evaluation of the airway, heart, and lungs. Vital signs are reviewed, and auscultation of the heart and lungs is performed in a standard fashion. Peripheral pulses are palpated and compared.

Careful examination of the airway allows identification of patients at increased risk for difficult mask ventilation or difficult tracheal intubation. No single examination or sign is adequate to identify all patients at risk for difficult tracheal intubation. Among the factors that are assessed are: mouth opening; neck motion; size, shape, and abnormalities of the teeth; relative size of tongue and oropharynx; and distance from the tip of the chin to the anterior aspect of the thyroid cartilage or hyoid bone.

7. **What diagnostic studies are necessary to complete the preanesthesia assessment?**

There is no absolute group of studies that are indicated in all patients. The choice of additional testing is guided by the history and physical examination. Typically, a hemoglobin or hematocrit, serum electrolytes, blood urea nitrogen (BUN), and creatinine are obtained for patients with cardiac disease. For patients who have no history of bleeding problems, there is no benefit from obtaining preoperative coagulation tests.

An electrocardiogram (ECG) should be obtained for patients with a history of cardiac disease. The ECG can identify prior myocardial infarction, myocardial ischemia, cardiac dysrhythmias, and cardiac conduction abnormalities. Echocardiography can provide diagnostic information about cardiac valvular function and right and left ventricular function. Cardiac catheterization data delineate coronary artery disease, ventricular function, and valvular function.

A chest x-ray should be obtained if the patient has a history or physical examination suggesting pulmonary abnormalities. In the absence of specific signs or symptoms suggesting an abnormality, there is little benefit from obtaining routine chest x-rays.

8. **Describe the classification system used to categorize a patient's preanesthesia physical status.**

The classification system helps to identify anesthesia risk for patients. This rating system is not a risk stratification system, although there may be an association between higher physical status and anesthetic risk.

American Society of Anesthesiologists physical status assessment*

1	A normal healthy patient
2	A patient with mild systemic disease
3	A patient with severe systemic disease
4	A patient with severe systemic disease that is a constant threat to life
5	A moribund patient who is not expected to survive without the operation
6	A declared brain-dead patient whose organs are being removed for donor purposes

From: American Society of Anesthesiologists. Available at http://www.asahq.org/clinical/physicalstatus.html.
*This table is appended to the physical status for patients undergoing emergency procedures.

9. **What are the common risks associated with general anesthesia?**

- Nausea
- Vomiting
- Sore throat
- Hoarseness
- Pneumonia
- Awareness or recall of intraoperative events
- Organ system dysfunction
- Stroke
- Myocardial infarction
- Death

10. **What premedications are usually given to patients before cardiac surgery?**

Premedications can be divided into two groups. The first group are the medications that the patient has been taking before surgery. In general, antihypertensive (with the exception of diuretics) and antiischemic medications are continued into the preanesthetic period. The continuation of beta-blocker therapy preoperatively may be the most important of the patient's routine medications to continue. In patients with ischemic heart disease, beta-blockers have been shown to decrease the incidence of precardiopulmonary bypass myocardial ischemia, and lower the incidence of perioperative cardiac morbidity in patients undergoing major vascular surgery and other noncardiac surgical procedures. Angiotensin-converting enzyme inhibitors may be associated with an increased incidence of low systemic vascular resistance during and following cardiopulmonary bypass and are sometimes omitted on the day of surgery.

Medications aimed at reducing the risk of aspiration pneumonia may also be administered. These include H2-blockers, metoclopramide, and nonparticulate antacids, such as sodium citrate. An evidenced-based review, by the American Society of Anesthesiologists, concluded that there was insufficient evidence to recommend any of these therapies as a routine preanesthetic medication. Selective use, in those patients with risk factors for increased risk of aspiration pneumonia, may be beneficial, and is commonly used.

For diabetic patients, oral hypoglycemia agents are not given on the day of surgery. For patients receiving insulin therapy, there are several methods of managing insulin on the day of surgery. In the past, it was common to administer approximately half the patient's normal dose of intermediate-acting insulin on the morning of surgery. In current practice, it is common to omit all insulin therapy on the morning of surgery and to monitor serum glucose levels intraoperatively. Elevation in blood glucose is treated by titration of intravenously administered insulin.

The second group of preanesthetic medications are those used to reduce preprocedure anxiety. There are both psychological and physiological benefits from reducing preanesthetic anxiety. Preoperative anxiety, especially if it is associated with tachycardia, may be deleterious in patients with ischemic heart disease and certain valvular lesions (for example, aortic stenosis). A preanesthetic interview with an anesthesiologist has been shown to be more effective than sedative medications in reducing a patient's preanesthetic anxiety.

The classic premedication for cardiac surgery was a combination of morphine and scopolamine given intramuscularly. Scopolamine was used for its amnestic properties. A combination of scopolamine and diazepam has been shown to provide more amnesia than either medication alone. However, scopolamine causes dry mouth, which is uncomfortable for the patient, and can cause dysphoria or confusion that may continue into the postoperative period. Morphine can cause respiratory depression and may also lower blood pressure.

The most commonly used anxiolytic medications are benzodiazepines. This class of drugs reduces anxiety, causes limited respiratory depression, has minimal hemodynamic effects, and can produce amnesia. Benzodiazepines can be given orally, thereby avoiding the discomfort of intramuscular injections. In many surgical centers, preoperative sedation has been replaced with preinduction sedation given in the preoperative area and then supplemented, as needed, in the operating room. Preinduction sedation, given intravenously, typically includes a benzodiazepine and an opioid. This timing of the sedation has the advantage of withholding sedative medications until the patient is being monitored by the anesthesiologist.

11. Describe the nondepolarizing neuromuscular blocking agents and their hemodynamic side effects.

Nondepolarizing neuromuscular blocking agents		
	Predominant Route of Elimination	Hemodynamic Side Effects
Short Duration:		
Mivacurium	Plasma cholinesterase	Mild histamine release, possible decreased BP
Intermediate Duration:		
Atracurium	Hofmann degradation (nonenzymatic)	Mild histamine release, possible decreased BP
Cisatracurium	Hofmann degradation (nonenzymatic)	None
Rocuronium	Hepatic	None
Vecuronium	Hepatic	None
Long Duration:		
Pancuronium	Renal	Increased heart rate

12. What are the basic intraoperative anesthesia monitoring tools for cardiac surgery patients?
- ECG monitoring
- Continuous pulse oximetry
- Intraarterial line for blood pressure monitoring
- Body temperature monitoring
- Pulmonary artery (PA) catheter monitoring

13. What data are obtained using a pulmonary artery catheter?

Using a multilumen pulmonary artery (PA) catheter will allow for the measurement of right atrial, pulmonary artery, and pulmonary artery occlusion pressures. A PA catheter also permits the measurement of cardiac output using the thermal dilution technique. Using the data obtained with a PA catheter, a variety of derived hemodynamic variables can be calculated (cardiac index, systemic and pulmonary vascular resistance, stroke volume, stroke volume index, stroke work index).

Mixed venous oxygen saturation can be continuously monitored using a PA catheter equipped with a fiberoptic sensor. Mixed venous oxygen saturation provides a global (whole body) assessment of the balance between oxygen delivery and oxygen consumption. The oxygen delivery is determined by cardiac output, arterial partial pressure of oxygen (PaO_2), oxyhemoglobin saturations, and hemoglobin concentration. When other factors remain constant, the mixed venous oxygen concentration will vary directly with cardiac output. The normal mixed venous oxygen saturation is 75%; saturation below 50% to 60% suggests

inadequate oxygen delivery to meet oxygen demands. Just as there are no con-
clusive data showing that use of a pulmonary artery catheter is associated with
a better outcome in cardiac surgical patients, the addition of mixed venous
oximetry has not been shown to improve outcome.

14. **Describe conditions in which the left ventricular end-diastolic pressure (LVEDP) may differ from the pulmonary occlusion pressure (POP).**

   - Pulmonary artery occlusion pressure > left ventricular end-diastolic pressure
   - Mitral stenosis
   - Increased airway pressure
   - Left atrial myxoma
   - Pulmonary artery occlusion pressure < left ventricular end-diastolic pressure
   - Noncompliant ventricle
   - LVEDP > 25 mm Hg
   - Aortic insufficiency
   - Pulmonary artery diastolic pressure > pulmonary artery occlusion pressure
   - Increased pulmonary vascular resistance
   - Noncardiac pulmonary edema
   - Tachycardia

15. **What is the role of transesophageal echocardiography (TEE) in monitoring patients undergoing cardiac surgery?**

   Transesophageal echocardiography has become an important monitor during
   anesthesia for cardiac surgery. Currently TEE is the most sensitive monitor for
   myocardial ischemia. The appearance of new regional wall motion abnormalities in the left ventricle is generally presumed to represent areas of myocardial
   ischemia. The cost of TEE equipment and the lack of automation in the detection of changes in regional wall motion and overall ventricular function are disadvantages of its use as a monitor. TEE also requires an experienced operator to
   perform the study. TEE examination may distract the anesthesiologist from
   other monitoring tasks. In the postoperative period, TEE is a useful diagnostic
   tool, but is not practical for monitoring purposes.

   Transesophageal echocardiography is an important diagnostic tool during
   valve replacement or repair surgery. It allows for the assessment of valve pathology at the beginning of the procedure, sometimes helping the surgeon decide
   whether a valvular lesion needs to be addressed during coronary artery bypass
   surgery (for example, judging the severity of mitral regurgitation). After completion of the surgical procedure, TEE is an important diagnostic tool used to
   judge the integrity of valve replacement or repair.

16. **What are some of the potential complications associated with the passage of the TEE probe?**

   Like all invasive procedures, TEE is not risk-free. The placement of the probe,
   which is the size of a gastroscope, into the esophagus can be associated with
   pharyngeal, esophageal, and gastric injury. Thermal injury to the esophagus or

stomach can also occur (rarely) from the heat generated at the tip of the probe by the energy of the sound waves.

17. What type of monitoring may be used to assess awareness during anesthesia?

Bispectral index (BIS) monitoring uses a processed EEG to evaluate unconsciousness. The BIS monitor subjects the signal from a single-lead frontal EEG to processing that includes analysis of power and frequency. The analysis also includes information about beta-activation, burst suppression, and coherence. An empirically derived algorithm is used to calculate a dimensionless number between 0 and 100. Awareness and recall of events are usually absent with a BIS number below 60.

18. What is the role of opioids in the intraoperative management of cardiac surgery patients?

Opioids are a class of medications that stimulate specific opioid receptors in the brain and spinal cord. Their primary effect is to produce analgesia. Agents currently used in anesthesia practice include morphine, meperidine, hydromorphone, alfentanil, fentanyl, remifentanil, and sufentanil. Of these, fentanyl and sufentanil are the most commonly used agents for cardiac anesthesia. Opioids are not complete anesthetics. They are unreliable in assuring unconsciousness and amnesia, and they do not produce muscle relaxation.

The limited hemodynamic effects of opioids make them very useful in patients with cardiac disease. Opioids do not cause tachycardia; in fact they frequently will be associated with a reduction in heart rate. In general, with the exception of morphine, their effect on blood pressure is minimal. Morphine administration can cause histamine release, leading to hypotension secondary to vasodilatation. Opioids, except for meperidine, do not cause myocardial depression. Opioids are well tolerated, even in high doses, in patients with limited cardiac reserve. They are also very effective at blunting the sympathetic nervous system response to noxious stimuli.

High doses of opioids can cause chest wall rigidity, which can make mask ventilation difficult. The administration of a neuromuscular blocking agent will resolve the chest wall rigidity. Chest wall rigidity, with associated respiratory distress, has been described in patients recovering from an opioid-based anesthetic, but this is not common. The opioid antagonist naloxone will also reverse chest wall rigidity.

Opioids produce dose-dependent respiratory depression. A high-dose opioid anesthetic will necessitate a period of postoperative mechanical ventilation, until the opioid level in the blood has been reduced below the respiratory depression threshold by redistribution and metabolism. The duration of postoperative respiratory depression will depend on the total dose of opioid administered, the additive effects from other medications, and the rate at which the patient is able to metabolize the medications. Older patients will often have a more prolonged recovery, while patients who are opioid-tolerant will recover faster. Despite this potential disadvantage, a high-dose narcotic anesthetic may be the best choice for patients who have very poor ventricular function or who are hemodynamically unstable before the induction of anesthesia (for example, patients in cardiogenic shock). Because this technique may not reliably produce unconsciousness and amnesia, supplementation of the anesthetic with a benzodiazepine or volatile inhaled anesthetic agent is common.

19. What is the physiological effect of benzodiazepines?

Benzodiazepines produce unconsciousness and amnesia, but do not produce analgesia. As a single agent, benzodiazepines will not blunt the sympathetic nervous system (SNS) response to noxious stimuli. The agents used during anesthesia include: diazepam, lorazepam, and midazolam. Benzodiazepines, when given alone, cause little change in hemodynamic parameters. There may be a mild decrease in blood pressure, with midazolam > lorazepam > diazepam. Benzodiazepines cause little change in heart rate, and ventricular function is preserved. The duration of action for these agents is: diazepam > lorazepam > midazolam.

Benzodiazepines can be used to induce anesthesia. As an induction agent, a benzodiazepine will induce unconsciousness and amnesia without associated chest wall rigidity. An opioid is commonly administered after the patient is unconscious to blunt the response to noxious stimuli; however, the combination of a benzodiazepine and an opioid can result in vasodilatation, with the potential for hypotension. Careful titration and timing of the benzodiazepine and opioids will lead to a hemodynamically stable induction.

In higher doses, benzodiazepines also can cause respiratory depression, but this effect is less than that with opioids. Because of their ability to produce amnesia, they are frequently used as a supplement to other anesthetic agents.

20. What is thiopental?

Thiopental, an ultra-short-acting barbiturate, can rapidly induce unconsciousness. Because of its high lipid solubility and rapid redistribution, the effect of a single dose of thiopental is brief. Administration of an induction dose of thiopental is associated with a decrease in blood pressure, secondary to peripheral vasodilatation. Because thiopental does not depress baroreceptor function, the decrease in blood pressure is typically associated with an increase in heart rate. Venodilatation can lead to a decrease in venous return to the heart, which leads to a decrease in cardiac output. The increase in heart rate will partially offset the decrease in cardiac output. Thiopental in vitro has negative inotropic effects. The decrease in blood pressure associated with the administration of thiopental is exaggerated in patients who are hypovolemic and in those who have poor ventricular function. Thiopental does not blunt the SNS response to laryngoscopy and intubation.

21. What is propofol?

Propofol is a nonbarbiturate short-acting sedative–hypnotic agent. It will also rapidly induce unconsciousness, with rapid recovery. Propofol decreases systemic vascular resistance more than thiopental. It has little effect on heart rate. Therefore the decline in blood pressure following administration of an induction dose of propofol is greater than that seen with thiopental. Propofol has negative inotropic effects. The decrease in blood pressure seen with propofol is greater in patients who are hypovolemic and those with poor ventricular function. Propofol can be administered by continuous infusion with rapid recovery with minimal residual ("hangover") effect following its discontinuation. Propofol infusion can be used as part of an anesthetic technique to allow rapid recovery and tracheal extubation. A propofol infusion can also be used for sedation in the intensive care unit.

22. What is ketamine?

Ketamine is a phencyclidine derivative that produces a dissociative state of anesthesia. It can produce profound analgesia and unconsciousness. Ketamine does not cause respiratory depression or abolish airway protective reflexes. Ketamine causes sympathetic nervous system stimulation, resulting in tachycardia and hypertension. This sympathomimetic effect makes ketamine useful in certain circumstances (for example, in pericardial tamponade) but is a disadvantage in others, where an increase in heart rate or blood pressure is undesirable. Ketamine is a direct myocardial depressant, and in patients whose SNS reserve is depleted can cause hypotension.

23. What are the volatile inhaled anesthetic agents?

- Desflurane
- Enflurane
- Halothane
- Isoflurane
- Sevoflurane

24. What are the cardiopulmonary effects of volatile agents?

All volatile agents have cardiopulmonary effects. The effect on heart rate varies with the agent. Heart rate is decreased by halothane, is negligibly changed by sevoflurane and enflurane, and is increased by isoflurane and desflurane. All volatile agents decrease myocardial contractility in a dose-dependent manner. The comparative effects on contractility are: enflurane > halothane > isoflurane = sevoflurane = desflurane. Cardiac output, however, is preserved with desflurane and isoflurane because of the combined effects of preserved or increased heart rate and decreased systemic vascular resistance. All of the agents decrease systemic vascular resistance with isoflurane = desflurane = sevoflurane > enflurane > halothane. The blood pressure effects of the agents are the net result of changes in cardiac output (influenced by changes in contractility, heart rate, venous return) and systemic vascular resistance.

The volatile agents also have respiratory effects. In spontaneously breathing patients, respiratory rate is increased, tidal volume and minute ventilation are decreased, and the arterial partial pressure of carbon dioxide ($PaCO_2$) is elevated. Using the effect of the volatile agents on $PaCO_2$ in spontaneously breathing patients as a measure of respiratory depression, the relative respiratory depressant effects of the volatile agents are: enflurane > desflurane = isoflurane > sevoflurane = halothane.

25. What are some of the other systemic effects associated with volatile agents?

Volatile agents have only limited toxicity. They undergo little metabolism; their effects are terminated by elimination of the intact molecules via the lungs. Halothane can be associated with fulminate hepatic necrosis that can be fatal. This response is an idiosyncratic autoimmune phenomenon that is most common in patients who have repeated halothane anesthetics. Hepatitis from the other volatile agents is very uncommon. Transient hepatic dysfunction may occur secondary to alteration in hepatic blood flow by anesthetic agents, but may be difficult to separate from other causes related to the surgery. Enflurane may cause mild renal dysfunction secondary to fluoride ion production during prolonged use of anesthetics. Sevoflurane, in the presence of carbon dioxide absorbents, produces a substance (Compound A) that has been suggested to cause renal dysfunction; however, this issue remains controversial. All volatile agents can trigger malignant hyperthermia in susceptible individuals.

26. What is the anesthesia goal for the patient undergoing cardiac surgery?

A common goal is to maintain hemodynamic stability and provide a smooth transition from consciousness into the anesthetic state and then continuing hemodynamic stability and unconsciousness throughout the procedure.

27. Describe the hemodynamic goals for selected cardiac pathology when undergoing cardiac surgery.

Hemodynamic goals during anesthesia for patient with cardiac disease

Cardiac Condition	Preload (Intravascular Volume)	Afterload	Heart Rate and Rhythm
Coronary artery disease	Maintain to slightly lower	Maintain to maintain blood pressure and coronary perfusion pressure	Decrease, slower heart rate better; avoid tachycardia
Aortic stenosis	Maintain full	Maintain; prevent vasodilatation and hypotension	Avoid tachycardia; maintain sinus rhythm if possible
Aortic regurgitation	Maintain to slightly increased	Decrease to decrease regurgitant flow	Maintain to mild increase
Mitral stenosis	Maintain adequate to preserve LV filling	Maintain; avoid increased pulmonary resistance	Prevent tachycardia, maintain sinus rhythm if possible
Mitral regurgitation	Maintain	Decrease to decrease regurgitant flow	Maintain to mild increase

28. **What are the three periods of anesthesia?**

- Induction
- Maintenance
- Recovery

    For surgical procedures that involve the use of cardiopulmonary bypass (CPB), the maintenance period can be separated into the pre-CPB, CPB, and post-CPB periods.

29. **How is anticoagulation managed intraoperatively?**

Anticoagulation is required for all procedures involving cardiopulmonary bypass and for coronary artery bypass grafting (CABG) without CPB (off-pump CABG). Anticoagulation before CPB is achieved with administration of intravenous heparin in a dose of 300 to 400 units/kg. The effect of the heparin is monitored by measuring the activated clotting time (ACT), a modified whole blood clotting test that can be performed in the operating room. The normal ACT is in the range of 80 to 120 seconds. An adequate level of anticoagulation for CPB will have an ACT greater than 480 seconds. The level of anticoagulation used for off-pump CABG can vary among surgeons. Some surgeons will use similar levels of anticoagulation for on-pump and off-pump CABG; others will use lower levels of anticoagulation for off-pump CABG. Cardiopulmonary bypass is initiated once anticoagulation is appropriate and the various perfusion cannulas are in place.

30. **How is systemic hypothermia managed in the patient on cardiopulmonary bypass?**

If systemic hypothermia is used, the patient will need to be rewarmed in preparation for separation from CPB. Regions of the body cool and warm at different rates, depending on their mass and blood flow. The vessel-rich organs (brain, heart, kidney, lung, liver) will warm faster than the muscle group, which in turn will warm faster than fat. Bladder or rectal temperature is monitored as an assessment of the temperature in more peripheral sites. This is important to assure adequate rewarming. If a patient is warmed only until their core temperature (blood, esophageal, nasopharyngeal temperature) has reached 37° C (98.6° F) but their more peripheral tissues are still hypothermic (bladder or rectal temperature less than 36 to 37° C [96.8 to 98.6° F]), a drop in core temperature will result following separation from CPB. This occurs as the temperatures of the core and peripheral compartments equilibrate ("after-drop"). The after-drop in temperature can have several adverse effects. The coagulation system is impaired at lower temperatures, and this can lead to increased postoperative bleeding. Peripheral vasoconstriction, as a result of hypothermia, can increase left ventricular afterload, resulting in a decrease in cardiac output. Shivering can increase oxygen demands.

31. **What clinical parameters are monitored in preparation for a patient to be weaned from cardiopulmonary bypass?**

- Temperature
- Cardiac rhythm

- Acid–base balance
- Hematocrit
- Serum electrolytes
- Ventricular function by direct observation or TEE
- Peripheral resistance

32. How is anticoagulation reversed in patients undergoing cardiac surgery?

Following successful separation from CPB, anticoagulation is reversed by the administration of protamine sulfate. A small test dose (10 to 20 mg) of protamine is administered while observing for signs of an anaphylactic or anaphylactoid reaction. If no reaction occurs, the remainder of the dose is administered.

33. Which groups of patients are at risk for protamine reaction?

Patients with diabetes mellitus, who have taken NPH insulin, and patients previously exposed to protamine are at the greatest risk for anaphylactic reactions.

34. What is the treatment for an anaphylactic reaction associated with protamine?

Administration of protamine can be associated with histamine release, causing a decrease in blood pressure because of histamine-induced vasodilatation. This is the most common hemodynamic effect of protamine administration and can be treated with intravascular volume expansion and a vasopressor, such as phenylephrine.

Acute pulmonary hypertension with acute right heart failure and profound systemic hypotension is an uncommon, but very serious, side effect of protamine administration. The initial treatment of both anaphylactic and pulmonary artery hypertension–right heart failure reactions should be the administration of intravenous epinephrine. If there is not a rapid improvement in blood pressure and cardiac performance, it will be necessary to resume cardiopulmonary bypass.

35. How long is the period of mechanical ventilation in patients after cardiac surgery?

In most surgical centers, patients who have had cardiac surgery with CPB will have a period of postoperative mechanical ventilation. Multiple factors need to be considered in determining if it is appropriate to wean a patient from mechanical ventilation, such as:
- Normalization of temperature
- Hemodynamic stability
- Acceptable levels of chest tube drainage
- Acceptable PaO_2 on an FiO_2 (concentration of oxygen) of 0.5 or less

In addition, the patient should be awake, able to follow commands, and demonstrate adequate recovery of neuromuscular function. The respiratory rate, tidal volume, minute ventilation, and vital capacity should be measured during spontaneous ventilation to assess the patient's ability to tolerate spontaneous ventilation and tracheal extubation.

36. **What is the difference in anesthetic management of patients who undergo off-pump cardiac surgery procedures?**

Off-pump cardiac surgery procedures offer the advantage of avoiding the undesirable systemic effects of extracorporeal circulation. The anesthetic management will be similar to the pre-CPB anesthetic management described above. During the period of coronary artery grafting, the surgeon will manipulate the heart into various positions to allow surgical access to the coronary arteries that will be bypassed. This manipulation of the heart can cause significant hemodynamic disturbances, including hypotension, decreased cardiac output, cardiac dysrhythmias, and myocardial ischemia. The surgeon and the anesthesiologist need to coordinate their activities during the positioning of the heart to achieve a position that will allow the anastamoses to be performed with an acceptable blood pressure and heart rate. To maintain an acceptable blood pressure and cardiac output during this period, it may be necessary to administer additional intravenous fluids to improve cardiac preload or to add an inotropic agent to improve ventricular contractility.

The placement of the heart into nonanatomic positions may distort the ECG and make it of limited use for ischemia monitoring. The amplitude of the ECG signal can be greatly decreased when the heart is elevated for the creation of lateral and posterior coronary artery anastamoses. In a similar fashion, the nonanatomic position of the heart can make TEE images difficult to obtain and interpret. The mixed venous oxygen saturation, if an oximetric pulmonary artery catheter is in place, can provide information about global oxygen delivery and may provide reassurance that the cardiac output is physiologically adequate.

37. **Describe transport of the patient from the operative suite to the intensive care setting after cardiac surgery.**

The transfer of the patient from the operating room to the intensive care unit or postanesthesia recovery unit (PACU) must be accomplished in a careful and systematic manner that allows close monitoring of the patient's status to continue without interruption. At a minimum, ECG and invasive arterial blood pressure should be monitored continuously during transport. Additional monitoring, including pulmonary artery pressure, central venous pressure, and arterial oxygen saturation, should be considered. Monitoring of oxygen saturation is strongly encouraged in patients who have poor oxygen saturation before transport and in patients who have been extubated in the operating room.

Oxygen tanks must be checked to ensure that an adequate supply of oxygen is available for the transport. Possible delays during transport, especially if elevator use is necessary, must be included in the assessment. A full E-cylinder of oxygen has a pressure of approximately 2200 psi and a volume of 620 L of oxygen. At a flow rate of 15 L/min, this would be enough oxygen to last approximately 40 minutes. The volume of oxygen remaining in a partially filled tank is directly proportional to the pressure; therefore at 1100 psi the tank has approximately 310 L of oxygen remaining.

Medications needed for resuscitation and for the treatment of hypertension and hypotension should also be available during transport. Adequate intravenous solutions must be present during transport to treat hypotension associated with hypovolemia. An anesthesia facemask and a bag-valve manual ventilation device are also needed.

It is highly desirable to have all intravenous infusions, any infusion pumps, and the invasive monitoring lines attached to the bed on which the patient will be transported. Transporting the patient with rolling IV poles adds to the complexity of the transport and may distract the attention of the anesthesiologist from the patient.

Key Points

1. The three periods of anesthesia include:
   - Induction
   - Maintenance
   - Recovery
2. Clinical parameters that are assessed before weaning from cardiopulmonary bypass include: temperature, cardiac rhythm, acid–base balance, hematocrit, electrolytes, peripheral vascular resistance, and ventricular function.
3. Intraoperative anesthesia management may impact postoperative recovery.

Internet Resources

Virtual Anaesthesia Textbook: Anaesthesia for Cardiothoracic Surgery:
http://www.virtual-anaesthesia-textbook.com/vat/cardiac.html

Cardiac Surgery in the Adult:
http://www.ctsnet.org/book/edmunds

Bibliography

American Society of Anesthesiologists Task Force on Management of the Difficult Airway: Practice guidelines for management of the difficult airway: an updated report by the American Society of Anesthesiologists Task Force on Management of the Difficult Airway, *Anesthesiology* 98:1269-1277, 2003.

Broecke PW, De Hert SG, Mertens E, Adriaensen HF: Effect of preoperative beta-blockade on perioperative mortality in coronary surgery, *Br J Anaesthesia* 90:27-31, 2003.

Ferguson TB, Coombs LP, Peterson ED: Society of thoracic surgeons national cardiac surgery database, *J Am Med Assoc* 287:2221-2227, 2002.

Mangano DT, Layug EL, Wallace A, Tateo I: Effect of atenolol on mortality and cardiovascular morbidity after noncardiac surgery, *N Engl J Med* 335:1713-1720, 1996.

Practice guidelines for preoperative fasting and the use of pharmacological agents to reduce the risk of pulmonary aspiration: application to healthy patients undergoing elective procedures: a report by the American Society of Anesthesiologists Task Force on Preoperative Fasting, *Anesthesiology* 90:896-905, 1999.

Rosow C, Manberg PJ: Bispectral index monitoring, *Anesthesiol Clin N Am* 19:947-966, 2001.

Zaugg M, Tagliente T, Lucchinetti E, Jacobs E, Krol M, Bodian C, Reich DL, Silverstein JH: Beneficial effects from beta-adrenergic blockade in elderly patients undergoing noncardiac surgery, *Anesthesiology* 91:1674-1686, 1999.

Coronary Artery Bypass Grafting

Janice Jones

1. What are indications for coronary artery bypass grafting?

Coronary artery bypass is the construction of new pathways (conduits) between the aorta and coronary arteries beyond the obstructing lesion. There are multiple indications for coronary artery bypass, some of which are:
- Symptoms unresponsive to medical therapy
- Multivessel disease with or without depressed ejection fraction
- Two-vessel disease with depressed ejection fraction
- Compelling anatomy, such as left main coronary artery disease (≥50%), proximal left anterior descending coronary artery lesions (≥90%), or uneven distribution of vessels—left versus right dominance
- Unstable angina
- Previous myocardial infaction
- Complications from angioplasty
- Chronic stable angina, severity depending on exercise stress test results or number of arteries with significant stenosis

2. What are contraindications for coronary artery bypass grafting?

Contraindications for CABG are:
- Absence of open artery ≥1 mm after stenosis
- Absence of viable myocardium
- Coexisting severe noncardiac conditions with poor prognosis (for example, previous cerebrovascular accident [CVA], chronic obstructive pulmonary disease [COPD], aortic calcifications, severe peripheral vascular disease, renal insufficiency/failure, age)

3. What conduits can be used for coronary artery bypass surgery?

On-pump bypass and off-pump bypass use the same conduits. The internal mammary artery, left or right, has an approximately 10-year patency of 95%. The greater saphenous vein has a 10-year patency of approximately 50%. This is mostly related to intimal hyperplasia and atherosclerosis. Other conduits that can be used are the lesser saphenous vein, gastroepiploic artery, inferior gastric artery, or radial artery. To decrease the incidence of postoperative graft thrombosis, aspirin with or without Plavix is used.

4. **What are contraindications to the use of the internal thoracic artery as a conduit for CABG?**

- Diabetes mellitus
- COPD
- Previous chest wall irradiation
- Subclavian artery stenosis
- Ventilator-dependent before surgery
- Chronic corticosteroid use

5. **What are potential adverse effects of cardiopulmonary bypass?**

When a patient is placed on cardiopulmonary bypass, blood is circulated by a pump to other organs of the body independent of physiologic control (nonpulsatile flow). This allows surgeons to operate on a still, bloodless field. Cardiopulmonary bypass, however, causes a whole-body inflammatory response resulting in massive fluid retention, intercompartmental fluid shifts, multiorgan dysfunction, emboli, and hemolysis. These changes can cause cognitive dysfunction (1% to 5% possibility of stroke), renal dysfunction, pulmonary dysfunction, and bleeding.

6. **What are the criteria for considering a patient for on-pump versus off-pump CABG?**

This decision is determined by surgeon preference and skill.

7. **When would you consider referring a patient for off-pump CABG?**

Any patient considered for on-pump CABG can be considered for off-pump CABG, especially those patients with comorbidities, because these patients are at greatest risk for complications when cardiopulmonary bypass is used. Patients with low ejection fraction, prior CVA, renal dysfunction, COPD, aortic calcifications, or advanced age are at higher risk for complications after bypass, mostly associated with the deleterious effects of cardiopulmonary bypass.

8. **What are potential advantages to off-pump CABG?**

During an off-pump CABG the heart is beating; therefore the patient maintains a normal physiologic state during surgery (pulsatile flow). This can potentially result in less morbidity and mortality, which is associated with cardiopulmonary bypass. Patients who undergo off-pump CABG may require fewer blood transfusions, thereby reducing the cost of surgery and decreasing the length of time spent in the hospital.

9. **What are a few technical considerations during off-pump CABG?**

An off-pump CABG can be performed via median sternotomy or anterior thoracotomy. Complete revascularization can be achieved during off-pump CABG. The use of stabilization devices and apical conduits allows the heart to be manipulated to permit access to all areas of the heart. The stabilization devices isolate the artery and area to be bypassed while the rest of the heart continues to beat. Arterial shunts allow blood to flow through the artery while the bypass graft is being sutured.

10. **What are potential complications of off-pump CABG?**

One possible complication of off-pump CABG is the progression to an on-pump case. During manipulation of the heart, changes in hemodynamic stability may result in the need to place the patient on-pump to provide safe and complete revascularization. Hypercoagulability may be present because of the decreased amount of heparin used during the case. Bleeding may still be an issue because heparin is used. Dysrhythmias may still be present in approximately 30% of the cases; their cause is not known. Pulmonary complications may still be present because of the need for intubation and postsurgical recovery. Any potential complication associated with anesthesia can still occur, or any complication associated with coronary artery bypass surgery. Performing the surgery without cardiopulmonary bypass can decrease, but not eliminate, the risk of complications.

11. **What are preoperative nursing considerations for a patient about to undergo an off-pump CABG?**

While preparing a patient for off-pump CABG, the nurse should not only educate the patient about the procedure but also address patient expectations and questions concerning preoperative, operative, and postoperative phases of the surgery. Postoperative pain management should be discussed, and postoperative activity also should be reviewed, primarily ambulation expectations. Discharge concerns should be addressed, especially whether home care will be necessary; this way the nurse can begin to implement strategies to address patient needs.

12. **What are postoperative nursing considerations for a patient who has undergone an off-pump CABG?**

The patient should be extubated as soon as possible, in the operating room if possible. After extubation pain management and pulmonary toileting are of the utmost importance. Providing appropriate pain control will allow the patient early mobility and the ability to take deep breaths, cough, and clear secretions. This may be achieved with the use of patient-controlled analgesia. Cardiovascular status should also be monitored for hemodynamics (goal of cardiac index >2.0) and monitoring for arrthymias. Monitoring for bleeding is also important. Diet should be initiated once bowel sounds return. Fluid balance should also be monitored. Because there are fewer fluid shifts when cardiopulmonary bypass is not used, the use of diuretics is not as necessary.

13. **What educational topics should be reviewed with the patient after off-pump CABG in preparation for discharge?**
    - Incisional care
    - Postoperative activity should be reviewed, emphasizing the need for daily walking and the incorporation of an exercise program into daily life
    - Diet restrictions must be reviewed, providing a sample menu if available
    - Medication teaching
    - Lifestyle and behavior modification should begin; emphasize the need for continual follow-up with the surgeon, cardiologist, and primary care provider

14. **What are some of the factors that may lead to a poor outcome after CABG?**
    - Advanced age
    - Female gender
    - Left ventricular dysfunction
    - Diabetes mellitus
    - Renal dysfunction
    - Emergent procedure
    - Reoperation

15. **What are typical complications associated with CABG?**
    - Arrhythmias (atrial fibrillation)
    - Pleural effusions
    - Atelectasis
    - Incisional infections (sternal/graft site)
    - Neurological deficits (minor to major)
    - Mediastinitis

16. **What is mediastinitis?**

    Mediastinitis is inflammation of the mediastinum and is a life-threatening infection associated with cardiac surgery. It occurs in less than 5% of all cardiac surgery procedures.

17. **What are some of the risk factors associated with the development of mediastinitis?**
    - Use of bilateral internal thoracic artery grafts
    - Diabetes mellitus
    - Emergency surgery
    - Obesity
    - Prolonged bypass and operating room time
    - Sternal incision dehiscence
    - Delayed sternal closure
    - Postoperative shock
    - Reoperation following initial surgery

18. **What are the common manifestations of mediastinitis?**

- Fever
- Leukocytosis
- Pain unresponsive to analgesics
- Sternal drainage
- Sternal instability

19. **How is mediastinitis treated?**

Mediastinitis may be treated with antibiotics, but often a sternal debridement and removal of infected tissue is required. As a result there is a residual defect that may be filled by using a muscle flap. The muscle flap may be from the pectoralis or rectus muscle group.

20. **What medications are commonly prescribed when the radial artery is used as a conduit for CABG?**

Calcium channel blockers

 Key Points

- Left main coronary artery disease is an indication for coronary artery bypass grafting surgery.
- Atrial fibrillation is one of the most common dysrhythmia after coronary bypass surgery.
- Pulmonary complications after coronary artery bypass grafting may include pneumonia, pulmonary embolus, pleural effusion, and pneumothorax.

 Internet Resources

The Society of Thoracic Surgeons: STS Patient Information: Adult Cardiac Surgery:
http://www.sts.org/doc/3706

Cardiothoracic Surgery Network:
http://www.ctsnet.org

BIBLIOGRAPHY

Bedi HS, Suri A, Kalkat MS, Sengar BS, Mahajan V, Chawala R, Sharma VP: Global Myocardial Revascularization without Cardiopulmonary Bypass using Innovative Techniques for Myocardial Stabilization and Perfusion, *Ann Thor Surg* 69:156-164, 2000.

Buffolo E, Silva de Andrade JC, Brance JNR, et al: Coronary Artery Bypass Without Cardipulmonary Bypass, *Soc Thor Surg* 61:63-66, 1996.

Daniel J, Dattolo J: Minimally Invasive Cardiac Surgery: Surgical Techniques and Nursing Considerations, *Crit Care Nurs Q* 20:29-39, 1998.

Edmunds, LH: Why Cardiopulmonary Bypass Makes Patients Sick: Strategies to Control the Blood-Synthetic Surface Interaction, *Adv Card Surg* 6:131-159, 1995.

Morris DC, St. Claire D: Management of Patients after Cardiac Surgery, *Curr Prob Cardiol* 24(4):161-228, 1999.

Moshkovitz Y, Sternik L, Paz Y, et al: Primary Coronary Artery Bypass Grafting Without Cardiopulmonary Bypass in Impaired Left Ventricular Function, *Soc Thor Surg* 63:S44-47, 1997.

Newman MF, Kirchner BS, et al: Longitudinal Assessment of Neurocoginitive Function after Bypass Surgery, *N Engl J Med* 344:395-402, 2001.

Valvular Heart Surgery

Barbara A. Todd and V. Paul Addonizio

1. **What are the types of valvular prosthetics available for implantation?**
   - Mechanical
   - Biological (synthetic and human)

2. **What is the major disadvantage in using a mechanical valve?**

   The primary disadvantage is that anticoagulant therapy, which may lead to bleeding complications, must be used.

3. **What are the accepted recommendations for aortic valve replacement in patients with severe aortic stenosis?**
   - Symptomatic patients with severe aortic stenosis
   - Patients with severe aortic stenosis undergoing coronary artery bypass grafting
   - Patients with severe aortic stenosis undergoing surgery on the aorta or other heart valves

4. **What factors influence mortality after aortic valve replacement?**
   - Advanced age
   - Female gender
   - Decreased left ventricular function
   - Comorbid conditions

5. **What are the typical complications associated with aortic valve surgery?**
   - Stroke
   - Heart block
   - Bleeding

6. **What is the treatment for hypertension after aortic valve surgery?**
   - Volume resuscitation
   - Vasodilator administration

7. **What diagnostic testing methods may be used in the evaluation of patients with aortic valvular disease?**

   - Echocardiogram
   - Exercise testing
   - Radionuclide angiography
   - Cardiac catheterization
   - Magnetic resonance imaging (MRI)

8. **Identify factors associated with survival in patients with aortic regurgitation after aortic valve replacement.**

   - Decreased exercise tolerance
   - Left ventricular dysfunction
   - Chronic left ventricular dysfunction

9. **What are the surgical treatments for aortic valve disease?**

   - Aortic valve replacement
   - Aortic valve repair (selected patients with aortic regurgitation)

10. **What is the Ross procedure?**

    The Ross procedure, also referred to as the Switch operation, is replacement of the diseased aortic valve with the patient's own pulmonary valve. The pulmonary valve is then replaced with either a bioprosthesis or an allograft.

11. **What are some of the potential complications associated with the Ross procedure?**

    - Right ventricular failure
    - Aortic insufficiency
    - Bleeding
    - Rejection of the allograft
    - Pulmonic stenosis/regurgitation

12. **In a patient with mitral stenosis, what are the recommendations for valve replacement?**

    - Mitral valve area less than 1.5 cm^2
    - Symptomatic with minimal activity and at rest
    - Not a candidate for balloon valvuloplasty

13. **What are some of the potential complications associated with mitral valve prolapse?**

    - Mitral regurgitation
    - Infective endocarditis
    - Pulmonary hypertension

- Atrial fibrillation
- Mitral valve chordal rupture

14. **What are the recommendations for surgery in patients with nonischemic mitral regurgitation?**

- Patients with acute mitral regurgitation with symptoms
- Patients with symptoms despite normal left ventricular function
- Patients with moderate left ventricular dysfunction and dilatation

15. **What are the two most common microorganisms responsible for native valve endocarditis?**

- *Streptococcus viridans*
- *Staphylococcus aureus*

16. **What are the indications for valve surgery in the setting of native valve endocarditis?**

- Fungal endocarditis
- Acute mitral or aortic valve regurgitation associated with heart failure
- Annular or aortic abscess
- Valvular dysfunction and persistent bacteremia

17. **What are the indications for surgical intervention in the setting of prosthetic valve endocarditis?**

- Prosthetic valve endocarditis within the first 2 months of surgery
- Fungal endocarditis
- Prosthetic valve dysfunction associated with heart failure
- Paravalvular leaks, abscess, or fistula formation
- New onset conduction defects
- Gram-negative organisms with nonresponsiveness to antibiotics

18. **What is the goal for anticoagulation in patients with mechanical valve replacements?**

Aortic and mitral valve: target INR 2.5 to 3.5

19. **What surgical procedures are used to treat mitral regurgitation?**

- Mitral valve reconstruction
- Mitral valve replacement

20. **What are the advantages of mitral valve reconstruction?**

- Preservation of native valve
- Improvement of ventricular function

- Reduced need for long-term anticoagulation (unless indicated for other reasons)
- Decreased risk of endocarditis

21. What are some of the potential complications associated with mitral valve surgery?

- Bleeding
- Low cardiac output syndrome
- Arrhythmias
- Death
- Systolic anterior motion (SAM)

22. What is systolic anterior motion (SAM)?

SAM is a complication that may be associated with mitral valve reconstruction. The anterior leaflet of the mitral valve may billow into the left ventricular outflow tract, leading to outflow tract obstruction and worsening mitral regurgitation.

23. How is SAM diagnosed?

- Mitral regurgitation murmur on examination
- Echocardiogram

24. What is the treatment for SAM?

- Volume replacement
- Beta-blocker therapy
- Avoidance of inotropes
- Mitral valve replacement

25. What is the usual treatment for tricuspid valve endocarditis?

Antibiotics

 Key Points

- Mechanical heart valves require anticoagulation with warfarin.
- Low cardiac output syndrome may be associated with mitral valve surgery.
- Complete heart block may occur after aortic valve replacement.

Internet Resources

American Heart Association: Circulation: ACC/AHA Practice Guidelines for Management of Patients with Valvular Heart Disease:
http://www.circ.ahajournals.org/cgi/content/full/98/18/1949

The Society of Thoracic Surgeons: STS Patient Information: Aortic Valve Replacement:
http://www.sts.org/doc/3620

BIBLIOGRAPHY

Bonow RO, Carabello B, deLeon AC Jr, Edmunds LH, et al: ACC/AHA guidelines for the management of patients with valvular heart disease: executive summary. A report of the American College of Cardiology/American Heart Association Task Force on Practice Guidelines (Committee on Management of Patients with Valvular Heart Disease), *Circulation* 98:1949-1984, 1998.

Otto C: *Valvular Heart Disease*, Philadelphia, 1999, WB Saunders.

Cardiac Transplantation

Theresa Hollander

1. Describe the historical evolution of cardiac transplantation.

In 1967 Christian Barnard in South Africa performed the first human-to-human heart transplant. The recipient was a 54-year-old diabetic man with end-stage ischemic heart disease and *Pseudomonas* cellulitis of his legs. The donor was a victim of head trauma who was declared dead 5 minutes after cessation of heartbeat and spontaneous respiration. The recipient died of *Pseudomonas* pneumonia 18 days after transplant. Stanford University performed the first successful heart transplant in the United States in 1968. By the end of that year 64 surgical teams in 24 countries had performed 101 transplants worldwide. The patients died rapidly, and most of the teams quickly discontinued their programs. Since 1968 several important advances have occurred that have contributed to the success of transplantation.

During the mid-1970s Philip Caves from Great Britain developed the use of biopsy forceps for right ventricular endomyocardial biopsy to assess graft rejection and the adequacy of response to immunosuppression. During this same time period, Margaret Billingham developed a histologic grading scale for identification of rejection. In addition, rabbit antithyomocyte globulin was developed and introduced for enhanced treatment of acute graft rejection. These developments increased 1-year post heart transplant survival rates from 42% to 62% by 1974.

The definition of brain death was not legally accepted until the mid-1970s. Until this time the criteria for organ donation eligibility limited the availability of donor organs. The acceptance of brain death criteria and the introduction of cardioplegia and cooling techniques allowed distant procurement of organs.

Advancements in immunosuppressant therapy with the introduction of cyclosporine improved 1-year patient survival to 80%. Jacques Borel discovered that cyclosporine, a fungal metabolite, had potent immunosuppressive properties. By 1977 the University of Cambridge (Cambridge, U.K.) introduced cyclosporine into the renal transplant program. In 1980 Stanford University used the product in the heart transplant program, and by 1983 the FDA had approved the drug for organ transplantation.

The number of heart transplants has increased since 1980: 90 in 1980; 440 in 1984; 2500 in 1988; reaching a plateau of approximately 3000 in the 1990s. The plateau now is dictated strictly by donor availability.

2. What are indications for heart transplantation?

Accepted indications for transplantation include advanced heart failure (New York Heart Association [NYHA] function class [FC] II to IV), refractory angina, and recurrent life-threatening ventricular arrhythmias. Patients with advanced heart failure generally have systolic dysfunction because of underlying coronary artery disease or idiopathic dilated cardiomyopathy. Other diagnoses that may lead to heart failure requiring heart transplantation include valvular cardiomyopathy, congenital heart disease, restrictive cardiomyopathy, and hypertrophic cardiomyopathy. Patients may be dependent on parenteral inotropic medications or mechanical support devices.

Another acceptable indication for transplantation is recurrent or refractory angina not controlled by medical therapy and not treatable by traditional interventional or surgical techniques for revascularization.

Finally, patients with recurrent ventricular tachycardia or ventricular fibrillation despite optimal medical management and interventional management (pacemaker defibrillators and ablation) may also be candidates for transplantation.

3. What are contraindications for heart transplantation?

Because there are limitations in the number of organ donors, it is important to select patients who will survive and thrive beyond the transplantation procedure. It is also common that end-stage heart failure patients will have some end-organ dysfunction. Therefore frequently the evaluation of potential heart transplant recipients is best done when the patient is optimally medically managed and end-organ dysfunction can be better assessed. The following comorbid conditions have been found to have a negative impact on the outcome after heart transplantation and need to be considered in the context of the patient's heart disease:

Coexisting Systemic Disease: Diseases such as systemic lupus, primary amyloidosis, HIV infection, muscular dystrophies, and sarcoidosis may be contraindications to heart transplantation. The severity of the underlying disease at the time of transplant evaluation and the anticipated natural history of the disease process after transplantation need to be considered.

Pulmonary Vascular Hypertension: Hypertension may result in perioperative right heart failure and death. Assessment of the transpulmonary gradient (TPG: calculated by subtracting the mean pulmonary capillary wedge pressure from the mean pulmonary artery pressure) and the pulmonary vascular resistance (PVR: calculated by dividing the TPG by cardiac output) is helpful in the identification of risk. A PVR greater than 5 Wood units or a TPG greater than 15 mm Hg unresponsive to short-term and long-term treatment is associated with postoperative mortality.

Lung Disease: A forced expiratory volume (FEV_1) less than 50% of the predicted volume and an FEV_1/forced vital capacity (FVC) less than 40% to 50% of predicted may be significant contraindications to cardiac transplantation.

Renal Dysfunction: Patients who have a creatinine level greater than 2.0 to 2.5 mg/dl or a creatinine clearance less than 40 to 50 ml/min should be evaluated for intrinsic renal disease. Significant renal dysfunction is considered to be a relative contraindication to transplantation. Heart-kidney transplantation may be considered. However, 1-year and 2-year survival rates of heart-kidney recipients are 76% and 67%, respectively, compared with 83% and 79% for heart transplant recipients.

Liver Disease: Liver function test (LFT) abnormalities are common in patients with end-stage heart failure. If the LFTs remain abnormal despite normalization of systemic venous pressure, other liver disease entities must be assessed. Serology for hepatitis A, B, and C should be assessed. If the patient is actively manifesting hepatitis signs and symptoms, transplantation should not be pursued until the patient has recovered. With patients who have hepatitis C serologies, there are some controversies as to whether the patient should be a transplant recipient. Data suggest that short-term survival is not decreased in recipients who are seropositive at the time of transplantation.

Diabetes: In the past diabetes has been a contraindication to transplantation because of the long-term requirements of corticosteroids. However, common practice today is for rapid weaning of the corticosteriods. Considerations for these patients are the total end-organ burden, overall health, and quality of life.

Malignancy: Active or recently treated malignancy is a contraindication to transplantation, because immunosuppression places the patient at higher risk for malignancy. Patients with a remote history of malignancy have been successfully transplanted. Patients with a history of malignancy may be referred for transplant evaluation because of chemotherapy-induced cardiomyopathy. However, the patient must wait a period of time until considered "cured" of the underlying malignancy. All patients being evaluated for transplantation should be screened for cancer. This includes a rectal exam with determination of stool occult blood; women should have a pelvic exam, breast exam, and mammography. Men should have prostate-specific antigen levels.

Psychosocial Issues: Medical noncompliance and continuing substance abuse of alcohol, drugs, or tobacco are absolute contraindications to transplantation. Patients with underlying psychiatric disorders, cognitive impairment, or unstable social or living situations must be considered on an individual basis. Patients should be assessed for insurance coverage, especially outpatient pharmacy coverage, as the cost of immunosuppression is extremely expensive.

4. What does the heart transplant evaluation process include?

Each transplant center may have specific evaluation procedures. However, the evaluation typically includes the following:

General Information:
- Comprehensive history and physical examination
- Blood chemistry, renal and liver function panels, lipid panel
- Complete blood count, differential, platelet count, prothrombin time, partial thromboplastin time, fibrinogen level
- Thyroid function test (thyroid-stimulating hormone, thyroxine)
- Urinalysis
- Chest x-ray
- 24-hour urine for creatinine clearance and total protein
- Stool for occult examination

- Mammography*
- Papanicolaou smear*
- Prostate-specific antigen*
- Pulmonary function tests
- Carotid and lower extremity noninvasive arterial studies*
- Ultrasound of gallbladder*
- Consultation
- Psychosocial evaluation (psychiatry, psychology, and/or social work)
- Dental exam
- Nutritional evaluation
- Financial services

Cardiovascular Data:
- Electrocardiogram
- Echocardiogram
- Exercise test with determination of peak oxygen consumption
- Coronary angiography
- Thallium scintigraphy or positron emission tomography to determine viability
- Right heart catheterization with determination of transpulmonary gradient and pulmonary vascular resistance
- Endomyocardial biopsy*

Immunologic Data:
- Blood group
- Human leukocyte antigen (HLA) typing
- Panel of reactive antibodies (PRA) screen (% PRA for B-cells and T-cells)

Infectious Disease Screening: Serology for:
- Hepatitis B (HBsAg, HBsAb, HBcAb)
- Hepatitis C
- Human immunodeficiency virus
- Cytomegalovirus (IgM, IgG)
- Toxoplasmosis
- Varicella and rubella titers
- Epstein-Barr virus (IgM, IgG)
- Histoplasmosis and coccidioidomycosis complement fixing antibodies
- VDRL
- Stool for ova and parasites
- Skin testing for purified protein derivative (PPD) with control for mumps, dermatophytin, histoplasmosis, and coccidioidomycosis

5. **What conditions may increase morbidity and mortality after heart transplantation?**

The following is a listing of conditions that have increased morbidity and mortality related to heart transplantation:
- Coexistence of systemic illness with a poor prognosis
- Irreversible pulmonary parenchymal disease (FEV_1 <1 L or <50% predicted; FEV_1/FVC <40% to 50% of predicted)

---

*Only if appropriate.

- Irreversible pulmonary hypertension (transpulmonary gradient >15 mm Hg; pulmonary vascular resistance >5 Wood units despite treatment with vasodilators)
- Severe peripheral or cerebrovascular disease
- Active infection
- Irreversible hepatic dysfunction
- Coexisting neoplasm
- Irreversible renal dysfunction
- Active peptic ulcer disease
- Acute pulmonary embolism, especially with pulmonary infarction
- Active diverticulitis
- Severe osteoporosis
- Severe obesity
- Protein malnutrition
- Diabetes mellitus with significant end-organ damage
- Demonstrated noncompliance with medical regimen
- Current substance abuse: tobacco, alcohol, and/or drugs
- Psychosocial instability

6. How are heart recipients matched with potential donors?

A minimal prerequisite for allograft survival is ABO compatibility. A mismatch in ABO compatibility results in lethal hyperacute rejection secondary to preformed donor-specific antibodies in the recipient. Potential recipients with a history of exposure to multiple transfusions, multiparous women, and infants with congenital heart disease and multiple operations are at risk for having hyperacute rejection because of anti-HLA antibodies. Measurement of preformed antibodies is possible with the panel of reactive antibodies (PRAs), which measures both T-cells and B-cells. Patients with PRAs above 10% or specific antibodies may benefit from a prospective crossmatch before transplantation. Some transplant centers use medications such as Cytoxan during the pretransplant period to reduce the antibody load. Plasmapheresis and photopheresis have also been used during the pretransplant period to reduce the preformed antibodies. Simulect or other interleukin-2 (IL-2) agents may be used intraoperatively to reduce the possibility of early rejection.

The donor and recipient should be size-matched. The goal is to match the donor myocardial mass to the circulatory demands of the recipient. Stanford guidelines have established the safety of donor/recipient size mismatch as 0.8 or greater. A donor is considered marginal if mismatch is less than 0.7 or if the surface areas of donor and recipient differ by more than 30%. Before accepting an undersized donor heart, other considerations should be explored: duration of donor ischemic time, lean body mass, recipient's pulmonary artery pressures, donor heart hypertrophy, and gender mismatch (particularly if planning to implant an undersized female heart into an oversized male recipient). Undersizing should be avoided whenever possible but particularly in patients with elevated pulmonary vascular resistance and reoperative sternotomy in which there is a higher likelihood of rejection secondary to more transfusions.

7. **What are indications and contraindications for accepting and excluding donated organs?**

Criteria for **accepting** a potential donor organ include:
- Compatibility between donor/recipient blood types
- Verification of brain death and consent for organ donation
- Age <45 years or male >45 years with acceptable coronary angiography
- Female >50 years with acceptable coronary angiography
- Female >45 years at risk for coronary artery disease with acceptable coronary angiography
- Stable hemodynamics without high-dose hemodynamic support
- Donor/recipient size match within 20%
- Projected ischemic time <8 hours
- Functionally normal heart upon visual inspection at time of recovery

Criteria for **excluding** a donor organ include:
- Systemic sepsis or endocarditis
- Positive serology for HIV, hepatitis B virus (HBV), or hepatitis C virus (HCV) infection
- Active malignancy (extracranial)
- Coronary artery disease requiring extensive revascularization
- Previous myocardial infarction
- Irreversible ventricular dysfunction
- Intractable ventricular arrhythmias
- Structural cardiac abnormalities requiring extensive repair or reconstruction

Because of the critical shortage of organs, the donor pool has been expanded. Nonbeating hearts are included in the expanded donor pool because warm ischemic times are greater and there are higher rates of delayed graft function. When using an organ from the expanded donor pool, the risk of a patient dying on the waiting list versus the risk of dying from transplantation of an organ from an expanded donor must be considered. Whereas graft function may initially be worse and long-term survival less than if transplanted with an ideal donor, the risk of dying has been shown to be less than if the patient continued on the waiting list.

8. **Is there regulation and coordination of organ transplantation?**

In 1984 the National Organ Transplant Act was passed by Congress to improve the coordination and distribution of organs. This act established a national task force to study transplantation issues and to create the National Organ Procurement and Transplantation Network (OPTN). The primary function of the OPTN is to: (1) maintain a national computerized list of patients waiting for organ transplants, (2) ensure equitable access to organs for critically-ill and medically-qualified patients, and (3) guarantee that scarce organs are procured and used safely and efficiently. The United Network for Organ Sharing (UNOS) was awarded the contract as the OPTN. All hospital transplant centers, organ procurement organizations, and tissue-typing laboratories are required to meet the requirements of the OPTN.

Organ Procurement Organizations (OPOs) coordinate activities relating to organ procurement. There are 63 OPOs in the United States that serve in designated service areas. Their service areas do not overlap. The Health Care

Finance Administration (HCFA) of the Department of Health and Human Services designates, regulates, and sets the criteria by which OPO performance is monitored. OPOs evaluate potential donors, discuss donation with family members, arrange for the surgical removal of donated organs, and are responsible for preserving organs and arranging for their distribution according to national organ sharing policies.

The Health Resource and Service Administration (HRSA) maintains the Division of Transplantation (DOT). The DOT administers the OPTN and the Scientific Registry of Transplant Recipients (SRTR). DOT provides technical assistance to the 63 OPOs by working with public and private organizations to promote donation.

9. **How many heart recipients and donors are there in 1 year?**

Each year there are approximately 3800 new registrants for cardiac transplantation. The number of donor organs transplanted has remained somewhat constant at about 2300. The average waiting time has increased as the demand for donor organs has increased. The waiting time for Status 2 recipients (not in the hospital and not dependent on inotropes) has increased from 237 days to 382 days. Potential recipients die while waiting transplant because of a lack of organ donors. Ventricular assist devices have become the backup support to maintain end-organs as heart failure progresses. However, maintaining the potential recipient continues to increase the demand for a larger pool of donated organs.

10. **What is the process of matching donors with recipients?**

In the mid-1960s it was determined that transplanting a donor kidney into a genetically matched recipient improved graft survival. Consequently, several transplant centers began to share kidneys to improve outcomes. Methods for preserving and shipping the organs were successful. In 1977 the United Network of Organ Sharing (UNOS) improved the process by using computers to match donors and recipients. By 1982 UNOS was a national sharing network.

OPOs are alerted to a potential donor. Health care professionals may alert the OPO of a potential donor. The staff of the OPO has specific training and knowledge in counseling grieving family members about organ donation, assessing multiple organs for potential donation, and managing donors.

After the evaluation and management of the donor is in progress, the coordinator must place the organs. The federal government, through UNOS, regulates organ allocation. Coordinators register each donor with the OPTN, and allocation is determined through computer-matching by OPTN. Once a transplant center has accepted an organ, it is the responsibility of the coordinator from the host OPO to communicate with the coordinator from the receiving center to orchestrate and schedule the surgical recovery.

11. **What are the limitations of cardiac transplantation?**

Cardiac transplantation is limited by the scarcity of donor organs and by the short ischemic time of 4 to 6 hours. That is, the organ must be removed and be implanted within this 4- to 6-hour time frame. The procurement and implant process are orchestrated between the donor and recipient hospitals to reduce this ischemic time.

12. How are patients prioritized for heart transplantation?

Potential heart transplant recipients are prioritized according to their clinical needs, with the more severely ill patients given a higher priority. The UNOS listing status for heart transplant is as follows:

STATUS 1A
Inpatient at listed transplant center with one or more of the following devices or therapies:
  • Mechanical circulatory support
  • Ventricular assist device received within 30 days of being designated 1A status
  • Ventricular assist device received after 30 days of being designated 1A status but with a significant device-related complication
  • Total artificial heart
  • Intraaortic balloon pump
  • Extracorporeal membrane oxygenator
  • Mechanical ventilator
  • Continuous infusion of IV inotropes meeting the following criteria:
  • High dose of a single agent (dobutamine ≥7.5 mcg/kg/min or milrinone ≥0.5 mcg/kg/min) or multiple agents
  • Continuous hemodynamic monitoring of left ventricular filling pressure

STATUS 1B
Patients must have at least one of the following devices or therapies:
  • Left and/or right ventricular assist device implanted for more than 30 days
  • Continuous infusion of intravenous inotropes (whether at home or in the hospital)

STATUS 2
  • All other patients not meeting 1A or 1B requirements

STATUS 7
  • Patients considered temporarily unsuitable to receive a heart transplant

13. What are the immediate postoperative management goals for the heart transplant patient?

The immediate postoperative goals are the maintenance of graft function and the prevention of early rejection. The ability of the transplanted heart to generate adequate cardiac output in the early hours and days following cardiac transplantation is the primary determinant of post-transplant survival. Injury to the donor heart can occur at any time during the donor or implantation phase.

The donor heart may have sustained injury at the time of death (for example, myocardial contusion). Donor organ injury may occur after brain death, because management of donors organs offers many hemodynamic challenges. Injury to the heart can occur as a result of surgical manipulation at the time of donation or implantation. Ischemic damage and reperfusion injury also result in donor organ injury. Some degree of initial donor heart dysfunction occurs in 30% to 50% of transplanted hearts. Less than 3% of patients die from early graft failure. Improvement in donor preservation is identified as a major contributing factor to improved graft function.

Infection remains a major cause of morbidity and mortality. Approximately 25% of patients experience major injections during the first 2 months following transplantation.

14. How can perioperative and immediate postoperative graft function be assessed, and what interventions help support an injured donor heart?

Left and right ventricular systolic function is directly assessed in the operating room with a transesophageal echocardiogram. Inotropic agents, such as dobutamine and milrinone, are used to augment cardiac output and do not provide the alpha-adrenergic effects seen with epinephrine or norepinephrine.

Temporary diastolic dysfunction occurs commonly after cardiac transplantation. The hallmark of left ventricular diastolic dysfunction is an elevated left atrial pressure to produce adequate cardiac output in the presence of normal or near-normal systolic function. Diastolic dysfunction may occur as a result of ischemia and reperfusion injury, or may result from an "oversized" heart placed in a smaller pericardial space or from an accumulation of blood in the mediastinum that results in tamponade. Treatment may begin with nitroglycerin. Diuretic therapy may be useful. Afterload reduction with nitroprusside and then oral afterload agents is indicated. Milrinone may be helpful in providing inotropic support by reducing peripheral vascular resistance and increasing diastolic relaxation, thereby increasing cardiac output.

The right ventricle (RV) is particularly susceptible to injury and compensates poorly. Most transplant candidates have elevated pulmonary vascular resistance attributable to heart failure. Rarely, right ventricular dysfunction is a result of obstruction at the pulmonary artery anastomosis. Right ventricular pressure and pulmonary artery pressure should be measured in the operating room. Surgical revision is indicated if the systolic gradient is ≥10 mm Hg. If pulmonary pressures are normal or near-normal, management may include adding an inotrope and optimizing preload. If pulmonary artery (PA) pressures and the transpulmonary gradient are elevated, addition of a vasodilator and an alpha-adrenergic agent to support systemic perfusion pressure is indicated. Intraaortic balloon pumping may be considered. For PA pressures >45 mm Hg with severe RV dysfunction, inhaled nitric oxide should be considered. In the event of continued failure, a right ventricular assist device may be necessary.

15. Are rhythm disturbances a common problem related to transplantation?

No. Cardiac rate and rhythm are usually normal after transplantation. A total of 25% to 50% of patients develop sinus node dysfunction. Bradycardia may result in overdilation of the RV during a time when the RV is recovering from ischemic injury. The RV workload is increased because it is ejecting against elevated pulmonary pressures. Atrial arrhythmias may be the first sign of rejection.

16. What is the treatment of sinus bradycardia in the cardiac transplant recipient?

Treatment of sinus bradycardia may include atrial pacing. Drug therapy must **not** include atropine. Atropine is a vagus nerve inhibitor. Transplanted patients do not have an intact vagus nerve. Isuprel may be helpful in medically treating bradycardia. If bradycardia persists after 4 or 5 days, aminophylline or terbutaline may improve the rate.

17. How is the heart graft maintained after transplantation?

Rejection is one of the leading causes of death following cardiac transplantation, especially in the first 3 years following the surgery. Rejection is prevented through the use of immunosuppressant therapy and by careful monitoring of the patient. The patient is most susceptible to rejection the first 3 years following transplantation, and therefore must be monitored at frequent intervals. However, follow-up is a lifetime commitment by the patient and health provider team.

18. What occurs during rejection?

Donated organs are not identical to the recipient's genetic code, unless an organ is transplanted from an identical twin. Because the likelihood that an identical twin would donate a heart to the other twin is rare, a heart transplant recipient is usually different genetically from the donor. These genetic differences are recognized by the recipient's immune system. Consequently, rejection of organs occurs in at least one of three patterns: acute rejection; accelerated and hyperacute rejection; chronic rejection.

Acute Rejection. This usually occurs around 5 to 7 days after surgery. The tissue begins to develop inflammation and specific cell injury. Mononuclear cells infiltrate the donor organ accompanied by edema and reduced blood flow. Lymphocytes infiltrate and destroy the parenchymal and endothelial cells of the donor organ. Destruction of the cells and reduction of blood flow lead to rapid loss of function of the donated organ.

Accelerated and Hyperacute Rejection. If the recipient has preformed antibodies present at the time of transplantation or if there is an ABO antigen, hyperacute rejection follows. The antibodies on the endothelium fix complement, which attracts polymorphs, and destroy the endothelium within hours or even minutes. Assessing the potential recipient for preformed antibodies usually prevents this form of rejection. If there is a significant presence of preformed antibodies, a crossmatch with a potential donor will indicate if the potential recipient has antibodies that will specifically interact with the donor. Crossmatching involves taking the recipient's serum for determination of complement-dependent antibodies against donor lymphocytes.

Chronic Rejection. Cardiac allograft vasculopathy may be antibody-mediated, but typically no antibody is demonstrable and the pathogenesis is not understood. In heart transplant recipients the result is a potentially lethal form of graft atherosclerosis. The process usually is gradual, but may take months to years after transplant surgery.

19. **What is done to prevent major episodes of rejection?**

Clinical immunogenetics provides three major functions to reduce the risk of rejection:
- Tissue typing, which determines the ABO and HLA types of donors and recipients
- Detection of anti-HLA antibodies in the sera of prospective transplant recipients
- Performing a crossmatch, which detects the presence of antibodies that specifically bind to the cells of a prospective donor

The standard of practice is to avoid incompatible donor-recipient combinations. Hyperacute rejection occurs in patients with high anti-A or anti-B antibodies who are given an incompatible organ. ABO identification is mandated by UNOS.

Prospective heart transplant candidates' sera are crossed with a panel of common HLA types. The number of panels that the patient reacts with is quantified. If there are significant numbers of panels with whom the patient reacts (that is, ≥10%), then the patient is identified as a prospective crossmatch. Therefore before considering a potential donor, a crossmatch with the potential donor is required to assure that the patient does not have preformed antibodies to the donor organ.

20. **What causes anti-HLA antibody production to increase before transplantation?**

There are several clinical situations that may cause an increase in anti-HLA antibody production, including the following:
- Multiple blood transfusions
- Previous transplant
- Pregnancy
- Antiinflammatory disease (for example, lupus)
- Drug therapy (hydralazine)
- Infections
- Implanted devices (ventricular assist devices)

21. **What drugs are commonly used to prevent rejection?**

There are usually three drugs used to suppress the immune system:
- Calcineurin inhibitors (usually Neoral [cyclosporine] or Prograf [tacrolimus])
- Antiproliferative drugs (azathioprine or mycophenolate mofetil)
- Corticosteroids (methylprednisolone)

By interrupting the immune system at various phases of immune cell development, less toxic levels of drugs can be used.

Drug	Dosage	Side Effects	Drug Interactions
Calcineurin inhibitors			

Cyclosporine
Monitor trough
  levels; goal level
  dependent on
  how far out from
  transplant
Range:
  100-500 mg/ml
	IV: ⅓ oral dose
	  given in continuous
	  peripheral line in
	  1:1 solution of
	  D5W or NS
	2.5-5.0 mg/kg/day
	  given in 2 divided
	  doses q12 hr
		Nephrotoxicity
		HTN
		Weight gain
		Hypertrichosis
		Gingival hyperplasia
		Hand tremor
		Hirsutism
		Increased appetite
		Hyperlipidemia
		Headaches
		Cholestasis
			Inhibit metabolism:
			  erythromycin,
			  clarithromycin,
			  tacrolimus, sirolimus,
			  azole antifungals,
			  calcium channel
			  blockers, except
			  nifedipine
			Induce metabolism:
			  rifampin,
			  dilantin, phenobarbital
			Statins: cyclosporine
			  increases these agents
			  and increases
			  rhabdomyolysis

Tacrolimus
Monitor trough
  levels; range
  dependent on
  how far out from
  transplant
Range: 5-20 mg/ml
	IV: 0.01-0.02 mg/kg
	  continuous
	  infusion
	Oral: 0.1 mg/kg/day
	  in 2 divided daily
	  doses q12 hr
		Similar to cyclosporine
		  with less nephrotoxicity,
		  no gingival hyperplasia,
		  no hirsutism, less
		  effect on lipids and
		  weight gain
		Increased GI symptoms
		Increased glucose
		  intolerance
		Increased tremors
		Increased headaches
		Increased seizures
		  and alopecia
			Similar to cyclosporine

Steroids			

Methylprednisolone	500 mg after cross-
	  clamp removed
	125 mg q8 hr ×
	  3-4 doses
	1 mg/kg/day
	  tapering over
	  1 week to
	  0.5 mg/kg/day
		Pituitary adrenal
		  suppression
		Glucose intolerance
		Hypercholesterolemia
		Peptic ulcer disease
		Osteoporosis
		Hypertension
		Behavior changes
			Decreases action:
			  cholestyramine,
			  barbiturates, rifampin,
			  ephedrine, phenytoin,
			  theophylline
			Increases action:
			  salicylates, estrogen,
			  indomethacin, oral
			  contraceptives,
			  ketoconazole,
			  macrolide
			  antibiotics

Continued

Drug	Dosage	Side Effects	Drug Interactions
Antiproliferatives			

Azathioprine	2 mg/kg/day	Nausea and vomiting
		Stomatitis, esophagitis,
		  pancreatitis,
		  hepatotoxicity,
		  jaundice
		Rash, alopecia
		Arthralgia, muscle
		  wasting
			Decreases action: warfarin
			Increases action:
			  allopurinol

**Mycophenolate
  mofetil**
	500 mg increased to
	  1500 mg q12 hr
		Diarrhea, constipation,
		  nausea, vomiting,
		  stomatitis,
		  GI bleeding
		Leukopenia,
		  thrombocytopenia,
		  anemia, pancytopenia
		Rash
		Arthralgia, muscle
		  wasting
		Dyspnea, respiratory
		  infection, increased
		  cough, pharyngitis,
		  bronchitis, pneumonia
		Tremor, dizziness,
		  insomnia, headache,
		  fever
		Peripheral edema
		UTI, hematuria, renal
		  tubular necrosis
		Hypertension, chest pain
		Lymphoma
			Increases concentration
			  of acyclovir, ganciclovir
			Increases levels with
			  salicylates
			Decreases levels with
			  antacids,
			  cholestyramine

Protocols for immunosuppression vary widely; some factors affecting the protocol used are: the type of organ that has been transplanted, the length of time since the transplant surgery, the clinical presentation of the patient, and the preference of each transplant center.

22. How is rejection detected?

The patient is monitored for signs and symptoms of rejection. The most common symptom is fatigue. Examination of the patient may reveal hypotension, increased jugular vein distension, and the presence of a ventricular gallop (S_3).

Diagnosis of rejection is made by endomyocardial biopsy. It is usually performed via percutaneous internal jugular vein puncture with a fluoroscopic guided biotome.

23. How is cardiac allograft rejection graded?

International Society for Heart and Lung Transplantation: Grade of heart rejection

ISHLT Grade of Rejection	Slide	Description of Cellular Response	Treatment
0		No rejection	Routine immunosuppression
1A		Focal (perivascular or interstitial) infiltrate without necrosis	Dependent on grade and length of time since transplant surgery; some treatment options may include, but are not limited to: Maintaining optimal immunosuppression Increasing steroids Adding monoclonal (OKT3) or polyclonal (Thymoglobulin, Atgam) globulins Switching from Neoral (cyclosporin) to Prograf Adding Rapamune if chronic rejection by B-cells Using plasmapheresis or photopheresis
1B		Diffuse for sparse infiltrate without necrosis	

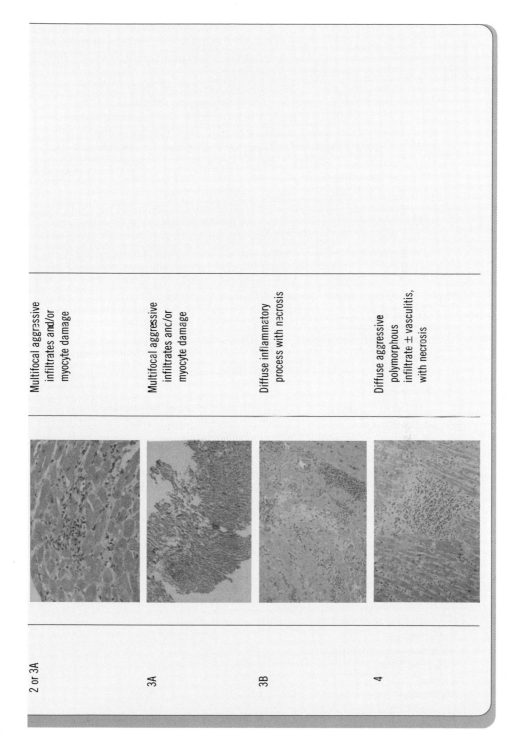

2 or 3A

Multifocal aggressive
infiltrates and/or
myocyte damage

3A

Multifocal aggressive
infiltrates and/or
myocyte damage

3B

Diffuse inflammatory
process with necrosis

4

Diffuse aggressive
polymorphous
infiltrate ± vasculitis,
with necrosis

24. What are the common infections seen in post-transplant patients?

Infection occurs in greater than two thirds of transplanted patients in the first year. It remains a leading cause of death. Occurrences of different types of infections vary at different times after transplant:

First month post-transplant: Immunosuppression is not high enough to incur opportunistic infections. The most frequent infections are related to surgical and nosocomial complications: bacterial and fungal wound infections, urinary tract infections, nosocomial pneumonitis (gram-negative organisms, usually *Pseudomonas aeruginosa, Klebsiella pneumoniae,* and other *Enterobacter*), line-associated bacteremias, and fungemias. The most common viral infection in this time period is herpes simplex virus (HSV) stomatitis, which usually occurs in seropositive patients pretransplant.

Early post-transplant (2- to 6-months post-transplant): Immunosuppression is the most intense during this time period. Patients are at high risk of developing serious opportunistic infections including cytomegalovirus (CMV), *Pneumocystis carinii* pneumonitis (PCP), invasive aspergillosis, disseminated toxoplasmosis, disseminated VZV (varicella-zoster virus) infection, and bacterial infections such as listeriosis. Tuberculosis and endemic mycoses can be reactivated.

Late post-transplant (beyond 6 months): Patients who have experienced rejections with increased immunosuppression are at risk for community-acquired infections. Tuberculosis, cryptococcal disease, reactivation of hepatitis B virus (HBV) and hepatitis C virus (HCV), nocardial infections, and herpes zoster are also diseases manifested at this time. Patients with chronic rejection are also at a higher risk for developing opportunistic infections.

25. What are the infection prophylaxis protocols used after heart transplant surgery?

- Bacterial prophylaxis: perioperative antibiotics (cephalsporins; if allergic to penicillin, use vancomycin)
- Fungal prophylaxis: trimethoprim sulfamethoxazole (TMP/SMX) for PCP
- Tuberculosis prophylaxis: skin test before transplant; consider isoniazid for +PPD (tuberculin) with epidemiological exposure
- CMV prophylaxis: oral ganciclovir for 3 months in CMV donor +/recipient −
- Herpes simplex virus (HSV) prophylaxis: oral acyclovir for 30 days
- *Toxoplasma* prophylaxis: TMP/SMX

26. What long-term complications are associated with heart transplant?

- Moderate to severe tricuspid regurgitation
- Hypertension and renal dysfunction
- Osteoporosis
- Rheumatological complications:
  - Hyperuricemia
  - Gouty arthritis
- Malignancy
- Hyperglycemia
- Hyperlipidemia
- Cardiac allograft arteriopathy

27. What is the life expectancy of a cardiac transplant patient?

Adult transplant recipients have a 1-year survival probability of 85% to 90% and a 5-year survival probability of about 70%. At 1 year after transplant, 85% are physically active and NYHA class I.

28. A 54-year-old man was the recipient of a heart transplant 1 year ago. He has had multiple acute 3B rejections that required an increase in his steroid dose, and on the last rejection he was treated with OKT3. He now is admitted with increased fatigue and increased shortness of breath (SOB). The chest x-ray indicates he has pulmonary edema. Right heart catheterization indicates: pulmonary artery pressure 58/22 mm Hg; pulmonary capillary wedge pressure 25 mm Hg; cardiac index 2.1 L/min/m². What diagnosis would be considered in his treatment?

Cardiac allograft vasculopathy (CAV). This complication occurs in 11% of transplant recipients in the first year. It is one of the more challenging problems following transplants. Diagnosis may be difficult. Angiography may help in the diagnosis. However, the diffuse nature of the disease may also not allow early visualization. Coronary ultrasound may be helpful. Early management of CAV may include optimization of the immunosuppression and reduction of the risk factors associated with CAV (hyperlipidemia, hyperglycemia, and hypertension). Sirolimus (Rapamune) has also been found to reduce the progression of CAV. Patients may be given a loading dose (varies from 6 mg to 15 mg; African-Americans usually require higher doses) followed by a daily dose ranging from 2 to 5 mg/day (African-Americans usually require a higher daily dose).

29. A 28-year-old African-American man was admitted with increasing SOB related to adriamycin induced cardiomyopathy. His history is positive for Hodgkin's disease, diagnosed 2 years ago and treated with chemotherapy. He is being evaluated for transplantation. Vital signs are stable: temperature 98.1° F; blood pressure 92/54 mm Hg; heart rate 110, sinus tachycardia; respiratory rate 24 on room air. He is currently on Vasotec 20 mg bid, Lasix 40 mg bid, digoxin 0.25 mg daily. He is 5 feet 11 inches, 128 pounds. Jugular venous distention (JVD) is present at 45 degrees with a prominent V wave and elevated to 12 cm of water. Lungs are clear bilaterally. The point of maximal impulse (PMI) is the sixth intercostal space midaxillary line. There is a loud S_3 and a grade 3/6 holosystolic murmur. His liver is mildly enlarged and palpated 3 cm below the right costal margin. Is there anything in these findings that is a "red flag" for transplantation?

Active or recently treated malignancy is a contraindication to heart transplantation. Patients with a history of malignancy should have a comprehensive evaluation to ensure freedom from malignancy at the time of transplantation or to assess the probability of malignancy recurrence after heart transplantation. Often it is difficult to assess with certainty the effect of chronic immunosuppression on disease recurrence.

30. A 24-year-old patient who is a new transplant recipient is receiving Neoral 250 mg q12 hr, CellCept 1500 mg q12 hr, and prednisone taper to 20 mg daily. The laboratory results are as follows: cyclosporine trough 558 ng/dl; Na 142; Cr 2.4; Cl 108; CO_2 24; white blood cells 16; hemoglobin 9.2; hematocrit 29; platelets 38. What adjustments should be made in the immunosuppression regime?

The cyclosporine trough is too high. The normal range is usually between 200 and 400 ng/dl, tending to be on the higher side for early transplant patients. Cyclosporine is nephrotoxic. Consequently, reducing the cyclosporine may help reduce the renal impairment.

CellCept inhibits cell division and nucleotide metabolism. CellCept can depress bone marrow cell lines and intestinal epithelial cells. Reducing the dose of CellCept easily controls side effects.

31. A 49-year-old African-American woman is a heart-kidney transplant recipient. She has moderate hypertension and is currently on hydralazine. Her anti-HLA antibodies are currently: T-cells = 46; B-cells = 0. Because of mild renal dysfunction, she occasionally needs to be transfused with packed red blood cells to maintain a hemoglobin over 9. In addition to increasing immunosuppression, what else can be done to lower her anti-HLA antibodies?

Hydralazine can increase anti-HLA antibodies. Perhaps using a calcium channel blocker for hypertension would be helpful post-transplant as calcium channel blockers may protect against cyclosporine-induced nephrotoxicity, perfusion injury, and delayed graft function. Calcium channel blockers may improve long-term graft survival by inhibiting T-cell activity.

Key Points

- Cardiac transplantation is limited by the scarcity of donor organs.
- Patients waiting for heart transplantation are prioritized according to the UNOS listing status as 1A, 1B, 2, or 7.
- Long-term complications associated with cardiac transplantation include: tricuspid valve regurgitation, hypertension, hyperglycemia, renal dysfunction, osteoporosis, gout, malignancy, hyperlipidemia, and cardiac allograft arteriopathy.

Internet Resources

Heart Center Online:
http://www.heartcenteronline.com

Medline Plus: Heart Transplantation:
http://www.nlm.nih.gov/medlineplus/hearttransplantation.html

BIBLIOGRAPHY

D'Alessandro AM, Hoffmann RM, Southhard JH: Procurement and short-term preservation of cadaveric organs. In Stuart FP, Abecassis MM, Kaufman DB, editors: *Organ, Transplantation*, pp 92-94, Georgetown, Tex, 2000, Landes Bioscience.

Eisen HJ: Left ventricular dysfunction after cardiac transplantation: etiologies, diagnosis and treatment. In Norman DJ, Turka LA, editors: *Primer on Transplantation*, pp 366-369, Mt Laurel, NJ, 2001, American Society of Transplantation.

Eisen HJ, Tuzcu EM, Dorent R, Kobashigawa J, Mancini D, Kaeppler HA, Starling RC, Sorensen K, Hummer M, Lind JJ, Abeywickrama KH, Bernhard P: Everolimus for the prevention of allograft rejection and vasculopathy in cardiac transplant recipients, *N Engl J Med* 349(9):847-858, 2003.

Fishbein DP: Evaluation and management of prospective heart recipients. In Norman DJ, Turka LA, editors: *Primer on Transplantation*, pp 323-326, Mt Laurel, NJ, 2001, American Society of Transplantation.

Haid SD, Kisthard JA, Anderson JA: Organ procurement organizations. In Stuart FP, Abecasssis MM, Kaufman DB, editors: *Organ Transplantation*, pp 69-89, Georgetown, Tex, 2000, Landes Bioscience.

Horvath KA, Fullerton DA: Heart transplantation. In Stuart FP, Abecassis MM, Kaufman DB, editors: *Organ Transplantation*, pp 225-243, Georgetown, Tex, 2000, Landes Bioscience.

Hunt SA: Historical overview of heart transplantation. In Norman DJ, Turka LA, editors: *Primer on Transplantation*, pp 321-322, Mt Laurel, NJ, 2001, American Society of Transplantation.

Kirklin JK: Immediate postoperative management of the heart transplant recipient. In Norman DJ, Turka LA, editors: *Primer on Transplantation*, ed 2, pp 352-362, Mt Laurel, NJ, 2001, American Society of Transplantation.

Norman DJ: Clinical immunogenetics. In Norman DJ, Turka LA, editors: *Primer on Transplantation*, pp 51-59, Mt Laurel, NJ, 2001, American Society of Transplantation.

Odim J, Marelli D, Laks H: Cadaver heart donor selection criteria. In Norman DJ, Turka LA, editors: *Primer on Transplantation*, pp 336-340, Mt Laurel, NJ, 2001, American Society of Transplantation.

Olyaei AJ, DeMattos AM, Bennett WM: Commonly used drugs and drug interations. In Norman DJ, Turka LA, editors: *Primer on Transplantation*, pp 99-113, Mt Laurel, NJ, 2001, American Society of Transplantation.

Parameshwar J: *Living heart donors—domino heart transplantation*. In Norman DJ, Turka LA, editors: *Primer on Transplantation*, pp 333-335, Mt Laurel, NJ, 2001, American Society of Transplantation.

Stevenson LW: The continuing evolution of donor heart allocation. In Norman DJ, Turka LA, editors: *Primer on Transplantation*, pp 341-344, Mt Laurel, NJ, 2001, American Society of Transplantation.

Stuart FP, Abecassis MM: Organ allocation in the United States. In Stuart FP, Abecassis MM, Kaufman DB, editors: *Organ Transplantation*, pp 60-63, Georgetown, Tex, 2000, Landes Bioscience.

Villacian JS, Paya CV: Infections in transplant recipients. In Stuart FP, Abecassis MM, Kaufman DB, editors: *Organ Transplantation*, pp 360-386, Georgetown, Tex, 2000, Landes Bioscience.

Yamani MH, Starling RC: Long-term management issues in heart transplantation. In Norman DJ, Turka LA: *Primer on Transplantation*, Mt Laurel, NJ, 2001, American Society of Transplantation.

Ventricular Assist Devices

Theresa Hollander

1. How do ventricular assist devices (VADs) assist the heart?

VADs help both the right and left ventricles pump blood out of their chambers and to either the lungs or the systemic circulation. A right VAD helps propel blood into the pulmonary trunk and then the lungs, while a left VAD ejects blood into the aorta and the systemic circulation.

2. Describe the types of ventricular assist devices.

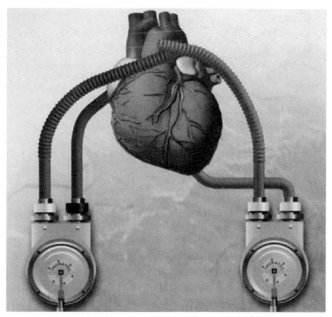

Thoratec VAD System. (*Reprinted with permission of Thoratec Corporation,* www.thoratec.com)

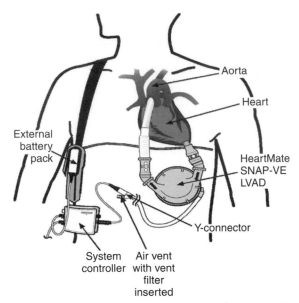

HeartMate VE LVAD. (*Reprinted with permission of Thoratec Corporation,* www.thoratec.com)

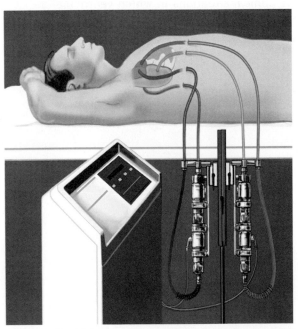

Abiomed BVS 5000. (*Reprinted with permission of Thoratec Corporation,* www.thoratec.com)

Types of Ventricular Devices

Thoratec VAD System	HeartMate VE LVAD	Abiomed BVS 5000
Used for postcardiotomy or bridge to transplant	Intracorporeal, electrically driven	Used for postcardiotomy or bridge to transplant as short-term device
Extracorporeal, pneumatically driven	IP model similar except driven by air	Extracorporeal, pneumatically driven
Blood sac surrounded by hard casing with valves on inlet and outlet cannulas	Pump implanted into preperitoneal or intraabdominal positions	Gravity-filled, vertically oriented pump
Vacuum to help fill VAD, compressed air to eject blood from VADs	Cannula inflow, through inflow valve into reservoir; pressure plate pushes diaphragm to eject blood through outflow valve and tract	Can be used for LVAD, RVAD, or BiVAD support
Requires anticoagulation	Driveline exits skin at RUQ and attaches to controller and power	Polyurethane valves
	Anticoagulation	Requires anticoagulation

3. **What are the clinical situations in which ventricular assist device (VAD) therapy can be initiated?**

   • Postcardiotomy shock
   • End-stage heart failure as a bridge to transplantation
   • Last resort for patients who are not transplant candidates

4. **What type of cardiac support does VAD therapy provide?**

   VADs can support right and left heart function. If support is provided to the left ventricle, often a VAD will not be necessary for the right ventricle, even when the right ventricle is severely hypokinetic. The LVAD will reduce the pressure in the left ventricle enough that the pressure difference allows the right ventricle to function effectively. The Abiomed BVS 5000 and the Thoratec can be used for both right and left heart support.

5. **What devices are approved by the FDA for clinical use?**

   There are currently five devices that are approved by the FDA for clinical use:
   • Abiomed BVS 5000
   • Thoratec Ventricular Assist Device System
   • Thoratec HeartMate VE/XVE
   • Thoratec HeartMate IP
   • Novacor

6. **What types of VADs are currently available for long-term use?**

There are currently four long-term VADs:
- The Thoratec Ventricular Assist Device System (Thoratec Corp., Pleasanton, California) is an extracorporeal, pneumatically driven system used as an RVAD, LVAD, or BiVAD system. It is used for postcardiotomy syndrome and for cardiogenic shock as a bridge to transplantation.
- The Thoratec Vented Electric (VE) is an electrically driven system.
- The XVE, a revised pump and system of the VE model, is an electrically driven system.
- The Novacor is also an implantable pump. These pumps are paracorporeally implantable systems; that is, the pumps are implanted into the preperitoneal area (a pocket is made using the rectus muscle) or into the abdominal cavity. These pumps are only used as LVADs and are used as a bridge to transplantation. During study protocols the VE and the Novacor may be implanted for destination therapy.

7. **What are common postoperative complications associated with VADs?**

- Bleeding
- Failure of the unsupported ventricle
- Mechanical failure
- Infection
- Pulmonary complications such as adult respiratory distress syndrome or pneumonia
- Thromboembolic events

8. **What is the Rematch study?**

The Rematch study compared treatment modalities for patients who had end-stage heart failure and who were not candidates for transplantation. The patients were randomly assigned to one of two groups: optimal medical treatment or Thoratec VE LVAS implantation. This was a multicenter trial.

9. **What are the main advantages of VAD implant?**

For patients who are candidates for transplantation and have been on inotrope therapy but are still experiencing a decrease in renal, liver, or other end-organ dysfunction, VAD therapy will help maintain organ function and improve their quality of life until an appropriate donor can be found. Patients have reported an improvement in their quality of life at 1 month after implantation and were satisfied with the implantation and optimistic about their heart transplant surgery. Destination therapy patients rated their quality of life significantly higher after implantation, as compared to the medically managed patients.

10. **When a VAD is used as a bridge to heart transplantation, are there any problems related to its use that place the patient at higher risk for post-transplant complications?**

With biomaterials such as VADs, indirect contact with the blood circulation elicits significant immunologic and thrombostatic alterations. Implantation of a VAD activates monocytes and T cells. There are increased levels of proinflammatory cytokines, changes in CD4 cells, progressive defects in cellular immunity, and increased risk for serious infection. The changes in CD4 cells result in polyclonal B cell hyperreactivity manifested by excessive production of antibodies, including those directed against human leukocyte antigens (HLA). This increase in anti-HLA antibodies reduces the number of potential donors available for VAD patients. The increase in anti-HLA antibodies increases the risk that the recipient may reject the transplanted organ. Therefore VAD patients with increased anti-HLA antibodies may require a cross-match with potential donors. The pretransplant cross-match may not be possible if the potential donor resides at a great distance from the transplant center or if there is insufficient time to obtain a cross-match. As a result, the donor pool available to the VAD patient may be limited.

Reduction in the formation of anti-HLA is related to the number of blood products that the patient receives before transplantation. Patients who receive fewer blood products, especially platelet transfusions, have significantly reduced antibody levels. Patients who receive leukocyte-depleted blood also tend to have lower antibody levels.

Elevated antibody levels can be reduced before transplantation. Use of pooled human intravenous immunoglobulin is one method that can reduce sensitization. When IVIg is combined with cyclophosphamide (Cytoxan, Bristol-Myers Squibb, Princeton, NJ), there is a significant reduction in antibody levels. Plasmapheresis and photopheresis are other therapies that can reduce anti-HLA antibody levels. The use of these therapies, however, is associated with side effects, such as infection, fever, rash, arthralgia, reversible renal insufficiency, and anaphylactic reactions.

11. **What effect does ventricular tachycardia (VT) or ventricular fibrillation (VF) have in patients with VADs?**

Patients with VADs generally tolerate malignant ventricular dysrhythmias. Patients have survived up to 12 days with an LVAD and continuous ventricular dysrhythmias. LVAD patients with ventricular dysrhythmias frequently experience lethargy, but remain fully ambulatory. LVAD-assisted patients may experience a significant decrease in device flow, mean arterial pressure, and central venous pressure. Despite the tolerance for VT/VF, it is important to make an early diagnosis and treat these dysrhythmias for several reasons. First, patients benefit from the early diagnosis and treatment of dysrhythmias as blood flow through the VAD is optimized. Second, treatment decreases the risk of developing an intracardiac thrombus, which may reduce the possibility of emboli. Third, correction of dysrhythmia decreases the potential of developing right-sided heart failure.

12. **Describe right heart physiology in a patient supported with a left ventricular assist device.**

Right-sided circulatory failure has been reported in 20% to 30% of patients with LVAD implants. There are significant changes in the right ventricular loading as a result of LVAD implantation. Some of these changes are beneficial and some detrimental to the function of the right ventricle. First, there is an increase in preload because there is an increase in cardiac output (VAD output). This increase in venous return and in pressure to the right side of the heart can result in septal "bowing" into the low-pressure chamber of the left heart. The septal bowing may result in diminished contraction of the right heart myocytes and reduction in right heart output. Second, usually right heart failure is related to left ventricular failure overloading the pulmonary vasculature and the right ventricle. Consequently, in the absence of pulmonary disease, the LVAD relieves the left side of the heart, unloads the pulmonary vascular bed, and reduces right heart failure. However, if there is an underlying intrinsic pulmonary disease in the setting of LVAD support, increased output and venous return to the right side of the heart with elevated pulmonary vascular resistance may increase the pressure in the pulmonary bed and result in right-sided heart failure. Finally, the LVAD increases coronary artery perfusion by increasing output and aortic root pressure. However, if the right heart is overdistended and the wall tension increases, then perfusion of the coronary arteries is reduced.

13. **How is right-sided heart failure treated in a patient supported with a left ventricular assist device?**
    - Volume loading
    - Inotropic support with medications such as Dobutrex and milrinone
    - Inhaled nitric oxide (INO) therapy
    - Pacing if there is no AV synchrony
    - Right ventricular assist device support

14. **A patient has been on the Abiomed BVS 5000 BiVAD for 4 days. How will one know if there is native heart function?**

The small peaks randomly interspersed within the large pressure waveforms (on the pulmonary artery waveform) from the VADs indicate that the native heart is beginning to eject out of the pulmonary valve and aortic valve. This can be confirmed by a transesophageal echocardiogram (TEE). If the native heart has recovered, weaning from the Abiomed and decannulation can begin.

15. **What are the exercise limitations associated with LVAD use?**

Physical therapy may be withheld if the LVAD rate is <50 beats/min, LVAD flow is <3.0 L/min, systolic blood pressure is <80 mm Hg, or intrinsic heart rate is >150 beats/min, with or without sustained VT or VF. The Borg scale of perceived exertion can be used to guide exercise progression with the goal of maintaining a rating of 11 to 13 on a scale with a range of 6 to 20. Upper extremity resistance exercises are delayed to allow sternal healing. Exercises that promote extreme bending at the waist should be avoided to decrease kinking of the cannulas. Bouncing, running, and jumping are prohibited because of the weight of the LVAD. Water activities are prohibited, although showering is permitted because of the VAD support components.

16. **What are important nursing considerations for a patient on a ventricular assist device?**

   - Infection prevention
   - Nutrition promotion
   - Rehabilitation
   - Patient education
   - Psychological support
   - Fluid status monitored

17. **Have the costs associated with LVAD implantation contributed to a reduction in the cost of treating heart failure patients?**

   Since 1970 the number of hospital admissions for heart failure has increased 10 times. In 1991 medicare reported $2.4 billion for hospitalizations and more than $10 billion for total treatment. Pharmacological treatment of class IV heart failure results in only 40% to 50% survival for 1 year. The projected first year annual cost of LVAD treatment is $204,797, which includes the initial hospitalization (accounts for 69% of costs), readmissions, and outpatient costs. As the LVAD emerges technologically, these costs will probably decrease. New technology is evolving, and future LVADs will be smaller, be completely implantable, and have a longer life expectancy. With continued success these devices may eventually be used not only as a bridge to transplantation but also as a long-term treatment option.

 Key Points

- Ventricular assist devices can support the right and left sides of the heart.
- The indications for ventricular assist devices include: for postcardiotomy salvage, as a bridge to transplantation, and as an alternative to transplantation.
- Mechanical failure is a major concern, particularly in the long-term assist devices.

 Internet Resources

CTS NET: Cardiothoracic Surgery Network: Frequently Asked Questions:
http://www.ctsnet.org/doc/100

American College of Cardiology Foundation:
http://www.acc.org/clinical/consensus/mechanical/future.htm

BIBLIOGRAPHY

Aaronson KD, Eppinger MJ, Duyke DB, Wright S, Pagani FD: Left ventricular assist device therapy improves utilization of donor hearts, *J Am College Cardiol* 39(8):1247-1254, 2002.

Andersmit HJ, Itescu S: Immunobiology of left ventricular assist devices. In Goldstein DJ, Oz MC, editors: *Cardiac Assist Devices*, pp 193-211, Armonk, NY, 2000, Futura.

Argenziano M, Landry DW: Management of vasodilatory hypotension after left ventricular assist device placement. In Goldstein DJ, Oz MC, editors: *Cardiac Assist Devices*, pp 111-120, Armonk, NY, 2000, Futura.

Catanese KA, Morales DLS: Outpatient left ventricular assist therapy. In Goldstein DJ, Oz MC, editors: *Cardiac Assist Devices*, pp 153-165, Armonk, NY, 2000, Futura.

Chen JM, Rose EA: Management of perioperative right-sided circulatory failure. In Goldstein DJ, Oz MC, editors: *Cardiac Assist Devices*, pp 83-101, Armonk, NY, 2000, Futura.

Christensen DM: Ventricular assist devices, *Advance* 4(15):17-19, 2002.

Damme L, Heatley J, Radovancevic B: Clinical results with the HeartMate LVAD: worldwide registry update, *J Congest Heart Failure Circ Supp* 2(1):5-7, 2001.

Dekkers RJ, Fitzgerald DJ, Couper GS: Five-year clinical experience with Abiomed BVS 5000 as a ventricular assist device for cardiac failure, *Perfusion* 16:13-18, 2001.

Farrar DJ: Physiology of ventricular interactions during ventricular assistance. In Goldstein DJ, Oz MC, editors: *Cardiac Assist Devices*, pp 15-16, Armonk, NY, 2000, Futura.

Frazier OH, Fuqua JM, Helman DN: Clinical left heart assist devices: a historical perspective. In Goldstein DJ, Oz MC, editors: *Cardiac Assist Devices*, pp 3-12, Armonk, NY, 2000, Futura.

Goldstein DJ: Intracorporeal support: Thermo Cardiosystems ventricular assist devices. In Goldstein DJ, Oz MC, editors: *Cardiac Assist Devices*, pp 307-321, Armonk, NY, 2000, Futura.

Grady KL, Meyer P, Mattea A, Dressler D, Ormaza S, White-Williams C, Chillcott S, Kaan A, Todd B, Loo A, Klemme AL, Picciane W, Costanzo MR: Predictors of quality of life at 1 month after implantation of a left ventricular assist device, *Am J Crit Care* 11(4):345-351, 2002.

Helman DN, Morales DLS, Edwards NM, Mancini DM, Chen JM, Rose EA, Oz MC: Left ventricular assist device bridge-to-transplant network improves survival after failed cardiotomy, *Ann Thoracic Surg* 68(4):1187-1194, 1999.

Hockman JS, Sleeper LA, Webb JG, Sanborn TA, White HD, Talley JD, Buller CE, Jacobs AK, Slatter JN, Col J, McKinlay SM, LeJemtel TH: Early revascularization in acute myocardial infarction complicated by cardiogenic shock, *N Engl J Med* 341:625-634, 1999.

Jaski BE, Kim JC, Naftel DC, Jarcho J, Costanzo MR, Eisen HE, Kirklin JD, Bourge RC: Cardiac transplant outcome of patients supported on left ventricular assist device vs intravenous inotropic therapy, *J Heart Lung Transplant* 20:449-456, 2001.

Jett GK, Lazzara RR: Extracorporeal support: the Abiomed BVS 5000. In Goldstein DJ, Oz MC, editors: *Cardiac Assist Devices*, pp 235-250, Armonk, NY, 2000, Futura.

Kasirajan V, McCarty PM, Hoercher KJ, Starling RC, Young JB, Banbury MK, Smedira NG: Clinical experience with long-term use of implantable left ventricular assist devices: indication, implantation and outcomes, *Semin Thoracic Cardiovasc Surg* 12(3):229-237, 2000.

LaPietra A, Grossi EA, Galloway AC, Colvin SB, Ribakove GH: Beating-heart coronary artery bypass grafting for left ventricular failure assisted by the Abiomed BVS 500, *J Cardiac Surg* 16:170-172, 2001.

Mancini D, Beniaminovitz A: Exercise performance in patients with left ventricular assist devices. In Goldstein DJ, Oz MC, editors: *Cardiac Assist Devices*, pp 137-152, Armonk, NY, 2000, Futura.

Massad MG, Cook DJ, Schmitt SK, Smedira NG, McCarthy JF, Vargo RL, McCarthy PM: Factors influencing HLA sensitization in LVAD recipients, *Soc Thoracic Surg* 64:1120-1125, 1997.

McBride LR, Naunheim KS, Fiore AC, Johnson RG, Moroney DA, Brannan JA, Swartz MT: Risk analysis in patients bridged to transplantation, *Ann Thoracic Surg* 71:1839-1844, 2001.

McCarthy PM: Implantable left ventricular assist device bridge to transplantation: natural selection, or is this the natural selection, *J Am College Cardiol* 39(8):1255-1257, 2002.

Morrone TM, Buck LA: Rehabilitation of the ventricular assist device recipient. In Goldstein DJ, Oz MC, editors: *Cardiac Assist Devices*, pp 167-176, Armonk, NY, 2000, Futura.

Moskowitz AJ, Rose EA, Gelijns AC: The cost of long-term LVAD implantation, *Ann Thoracic Surg* 71: S195-198, 2001.

Moskowitz AJ, Williams DL, Tierney A, Levitan RG, Zivin J, Gelijns AC: Economic considerations of left ventricular assist device implantation. In Goldstein DJ, Oz MC, editors: *Cardiac Assist Devices*, pp 183-192, Armonk, NY, 2000, Futura.

Mueller J, Hetzer R: Left ventricular recovery during left ventricular assist device support. In Goldstein DJ, Oz MC, editors: *Cardiac Assist Devices*, pp 121-135, Armonk, NY, 2000, Futura.

Pennington DG, Oaks TE, Lohmann DP: Extracorporeal support: the Thoratec device. In Goldstein DJ, Oz MC, editors: *Cardiac Assist Devices*, pp 251-262, Armonk, NY, 2000, Futura.

Ramasay N, Vargo RL, Kormos RL, Portner PM: Intracorporeal support: the Novacor left ventricular assist system. In Goldstein DJ, Oz MC, editors: *Cardiac Assist Devices*, pp 323-339, Armonk, NY, 2000, Futura.

Rose EA, Gellins AC, Moskowitz AJ, Heitjan DF, Stevenson LW, Dembitsky W, Long JW, Ascheim DD, Tierney AR, Levitan RG, Watson JT, Meier P: Long-term use of a left ventricular assist device for end-stage heart failure, *N Engl J Med* 345:1435-1443, 2001.

Samuels LE, Kaufman MS, Thomas MP, Holmes EC, Brockman SK, Wechsler AS: Pharmacological criteria for ventricular assist device insertion following postcardiotomy shock: experience with the Abiomed BVS system, *J Cardiac Surg* 14:288-293, 1999.

Shapiro PA: Quality of life issues associated with the use of left ventricular assist devices. In Goldstein DJ, Oz MC, editors: *Cardiac Assist Devices*, pp 177-181, Armonk, NY, 2000, Futura.

Sun BC: Device selection. In Goldstein DJ, Oz MC, editors: *Cardiac Assist Devices*, pp 27-36, Armonk, NY, 2000, Futura.

Thomas NJ, Harvey AT: Bridge to recovery with the Abiomed BVS-5000 device in a patient with intractable ventricular tachycardia, *J Thoracic Cardiovasc Surg* 117(4):831-832, 1999.

Management of the Postsurgical Patient with Cardiac Disease

Susan Baker Sample

1. **What are common pathophysiological presentations and early postoperative management techniques following cardiac surgery?**

   Patients usually arrive in the ICU with hypothermia and unreversed general anesthesia requiring mechanical ventilation. Patients may or may not require inotropic pharmacologic support initially. Patients usually show signs of peripheral vasoconstriction and polyuria because of hemodilution during surgery. The goals of initial patient management should include reversing the patient's hypothermia, controlling mediastinal bleeding, weaning from mechanical ventilatory support, maintaining hemodynamic stability, resuscitating fluid levels, and administering analgesics and sedatives as necessary. These are basic care techniques, and individual patient management may vary depending on the underlying disease process.

2. **What are common monitoring techniques in the initial postoperative period?**

   Continuous electrocardiographic monitoring: This is usually on a bedside monitor that normally displays one or two leads; the ECG is able to detect arrhythmias and to signal with appropriate alarms when necessary.

   Arterial lines and Swan-Ganz pulmonary artery catheters: These are hemodynamic measurement devices that are transduced at the bedside and provide accurate measurements of pressure when calibrated appropriately. Cardiac output measurements are determined using the Swan-Ganz catheter. Patient treatment decisions can be made quickly and effectively using these precise measurements for diagnosis and management.

   Continuous pulse oximetry: This provides continuous assessment of oxygenation status.

   Endotracheal tubes: It is important to assess for bilateral breath sounds with the intubated patient and document tube placement. Careful attention should be paid to ensuring adequate oxygenation and ventilation with mechanical ventilators. This can be achieved by monitoring arterial blood gas results as well as continuous pulse oximetry.

Chest tubes, urinary retention catheters, nasogastric tubes: These are drainage tubes that are inserted during the surgical procedure and are monitored for drainage frequently in the postoperative period.

Pacing wires: These wires are placed in the patient while they are still in the operating room following the surgical procedure. It is important to secure the pacemaker wires to the patient and to ensure a secure connection to the temporary pacemaker box.

3. **What factors should be considered when selecting inotropes and vasoactive drugs for use in the perioperative period?**

Various drugs are available to support patients with marginal heart function following surgery. Selection of these drugs depends on the individual patient's underlying disease, and treatment should provide adequate support of hemodynamics to the patient during this period. When selecting vasoactive drugs it is important to anticipate the drug's influence on preload, afterload, heart rate, and contractility. The table below provides a basic reference of the hemodynamic effects of common drugs used after cardiac surgery.

Hemodynamic effects of vasoactive medications

Medication	SVR	HR	PCW	MAP	MVO$_2$
Dopamine	↑↓	↑↑	↑	↓↑	↑
Dobutamine	↓	↑↑	↓	↑↔↓	↑↔
Epinephrine	↓↑	↑↑	↓↑	↑	↑
Milrinone/Amrinone	↓↓	↑	↓	↓↑	↓
Isoproterenol	↓↓	↑↑↑	↓	↓↑	↓
Norephinephrine	↑↑↑	↑	↑↑	↑↑↑	↑
Phenylephrine	↑↑	↔	↑	↑↑	↔↑

↑ = increased; ↓ = decreased; ↔ = no change; ↑↓ = variable effect.
Note: The effect may vary with dose level.

4. **How is pain control managed following open-heart surgery?**

Pain control is difficult to manage after cardiac surgery. Every person responds to pain differently, and therefore pain control methods vary according to patient needs. Recent studies show that elderly patients receive significantly less narcotic pain medications than their younger counterparts in the postoperative period. One pain control strategy that may be helpful is patient-controlled analgesia (PCA). This allows the patient to deliver pain medicine as needed without fear of overmedicating. Recent studies have shown that there is no significant difference in the amount of medication or the quality of pain control between PCA and nurse-delivered medications. Some patients respond better to being independent with their pain management. In some circumstances nonsteroidal antiinflammatory drugs deliver better pain relief, as seen in some cases of postoperative pericarditis. Overall, pain control needs to be individualized to the patient, as everyone perceives pain differently.

5. **What preoperative comorbidities increase patient risk of complications following cardiac surgery?**

   • Renal dysfunction
   • Chronic obstructive pulmonary disease
   • Peripheral vascular disease
   • Cerebrovascular disease
   • Morbid obesity
   • Hypertension
   • Diabetes

   These risk factors not only impact the incidence of negative outcomes but also increase the length of hospital stay, overall cost, and recovery time and affect the quality of life of the patient.

6. **What is low cardiac output syndrome?**

   Low cardiac output syndrome is a clinical presentation in which inadequate myocardial function results in decreased perfusion. Initially the patient attempts to compensate for this inadequacy with sympathetic autonomic response as well as catecholamine production. If the patient's condition continues to deteriorate, they develop advanced clinical manifestations that we usually associate with low cardiac output syndrome. These include:

   • Poor peripheral perfusion
   • Metabolic acidosis
   • Impaired renal perfusion
   • Pulmonary congestion

   Low cardiac output syndrome can develop as a result of inadequate preload, impaired myocardial contractility, arrhythmias, or elevated afterload.

7. **How is low cardiac output syndrome managed?**

   Patient management is individualized and aimed at treating the underlying cause of the syndrome. Management techniques may include:

   • Use of inotropes
   • Optimization of preload
   • Control of arrhythmias
   • Correction of possible noncardiac causes
   • Receiving a blood transfusion if indicated
   • Reduction of afterload if indicated
   • Treatment of ischemia or vasospasm
   • Use of IABP or LVAD if unresponsive to optimal medical therapy

8. **What is the role of intraaortic balloon pumping (IABP)?**

   The indications for use of the IABP are perioperative myocardial ischemia, postoperative low cardiac output syndrome, cardiogenic shock, myocardial

infarction with mechanical complications, and temporary support as a bridge to transplantation or placement of a mechanical assist device. The intraaortic balloon pump when correctly placed should be positioned in the descending aorta, just distal to the left subclavian artery and above the renal arteries. Inflation of the balloon pump should correlate with diastole, and therefore the balloon will deflate during systole. This mechanism provides afterload reduction and assists in perfusion of the coronary arteries. Absolute contraindications for IABP include:
- Aortic insufficiency
- Aortic dissection
- Severe aortic atherosclerosis
- Severe peripheral atherosclerosis

9. How is correct placement of the IABP assessed?

Critical assessment of the patient with a balloon pump should include:
- Monitor urine output hourly: if the balloon is not positioned correctly, renal artery perfusion might be compromised.
- Monitor perfusion of both upper and lower extremities: if the balloon is not positioned correctly, perfusion to the upper extremities via the subclavian arteries may be compromised as well as perfusion to the lower extremities at the insertion site.
- Monitor hematology studies: the mechanical action of the pump may destroy circulating platelets.

10. What are the indications for mechanical circulatory support in the postcardiotomy setting?

A circulatory assist support device would be indicated in those patients who have undergone a complete cardiac surgical procedure and are unable to be weaned from the cardiopulmonary bypass machine despite maximal support with medications and an IABP. This would include those patients in cardiogenic shock from a potential reversible cardiac insult or those who have continued deterioration despite maximal medical therapy. This device would be indicated in a patient who is unable to maintain a cardiac index >2.0 L/min/m^2 and a mean arterial pressure of <60 mm Hg. Eligibility for mechanical circulatory assistance should be considered if the patient is a suitable candidate for cardiac transplantation.

11. What is coronary vasospasm?

Vasospasm can affect normal coronary arteries, bypassed vessels, saphenous vein grafts, or arterial grafts. Diagnosis can be difficult to make, though general manifestations of this include: ST elevation in multiple leads, ventricular arrhythmias, heart block, and hemodynamic deterioration in blood pressure and cardiac output. Treatment for coronary vasospasm would include: optimizing hemodynamics (use of inotropes), administering nitrates (improve ischemia) or calcium-channel blockers, optimizing oxygenation, and correcting acid/base imbalances.

12. How is postoperative myocardial infarction diagnosed?

Diagnosis of myocardial infarction after cardiac surgery is difficult to make; however, persistent ECG changes are usually present. New regional wall abnormalities as seen on echocardiography can also be diagnostic of a new infarction. Cardiac enzymes such as creatine kinase (CK) or troponins are a poor diagnostic measure of myocardial infarction in this case, because postsurgical patients are usually oversensitive to myocardial damage. Persistently decreased systemic vascular resistance requiring vasopressors, prolonged inotropic drug support, or prolonged IABP use after surgery may also be diagnostic markers of myocardial infarction.

13. What is postoperative recurrent angina and how is it treated?

Recurrent angina is usually a symptom of ischemia after revascularization surgery. This can be caused by coronary spasm, diseased coronary arteries that are not bypassed, hypoperfusion syndromes, acute graft thrombosis, or anastomotic narrowing at the new graft site. Diagnosis of recurrent ischemia can be made using coronary arteriography, stress imaging, or calcium-channel blockers with coronary spasm. Treatment includes the use of nitrates, beta blockers, or aspirin or further revascularization.

14. What risk factors increase the possibility of stroke during or after cardiac surgery?

- Increasing age
- History of previous stroke
- Hypertension
- Diabetes mellitus
- Presence of carotid bruit
- Increased cardiopulmonary bypass time

15. What are common neurological complications following cardiac surgery?

Neurological complications can include:
- Central nervous system deficits, encephalopathy, and delirium (30% incidence)
- Seizures, neuropsychological or cognitive dysfunction (30% to 80% incidence), psychiatric problems
- Critical illness polyneuropathy
- Brachial plexus injury
- Laryngeal nerve palsy
- Phrenic nerve injury

Focal neurological complications occur in approximately 2% of patients undergoing cardiac surgery on cardiopulmonary bypass. Intraoperative neurological events are usually identified in the first 24 to 48 hours after surgery. Those events that occur later are usually a result of postoperative hypoperfusion/hemodynamic instability or atrial fibrillation. Overall, the etiology of serious neurological complications remains multivariable, and these complications occur in a small number of patients.

16. **What are common pulmonary complications following cardiac surgery?**
    * Atelectasis from the effects of anesthesia and extracorporeal circulatory support
    * Interstitial pulmonary edema
    * Cardiogenic pulmonary edema from hemodilution or underlying ventricular dysfunction
    * Pleural effusions
    * Diaphragmatic dysfunction resulting from phrenic nerve injury sustained during the surgical procedure

17. **What treatment modalities are used for pulmonary complications?**

    Most patients exhibit varying degrees of pulmonary complications following cardiac surgery; however, most of the complications are not clinically significant and do not prevent rapid extubation. Management techniques of mild to moderate respiratory complications can include arterial blood gas monitoring, prolonged weaning from mechanical ventilation, continuous pulse oximetry, chest x-ray, adequate analgesia, and pulmonary toilet techniques. Adult respiratory distress syndrome (ARDS) is uncommon after cardiac surgery, occurring in less than 1% of the patients, but it has a 68% mortality rate if it does occur.

18. **How is endocarditis diagnosed?**

    Endocarditis is diagnosed based on a constellation of clinical signs and symptoms as well as echocardiographic evaluation. The most frequent presenting signs and symptoms include:
    * Persistent fever
    * Fatigue
    * Rigors
    * Diaphoresis
    * Weight loss
    * Dyspnea
    * Embolization
    * Congestive heart failure
    * Delirium

19. **What risk factors are associated with the development of endocarditis?**
    * Valve prosthesis
    * Recent dental procedure
    * Rheumatic heart disease
    * Mitral valve prolapse
    * Intravenous drug abuse
    * Bicuspid aortic valve
    * Congenital heart disease

20. **What is the sequelae of endocarditis?**

Endocarditis can result in the destruction of the valve leaflets and the surrounding myocardial tissue, persistent systemic sepsis, and systemic embolizations of valve vegetations.

21. **What are the indications for surgery in patients with native and prosthetic valve endocarditis?**

The indications for surgery in patients with native valve endocarditis include:
- Persistent sepsis
- Moderate to severe heart failure symptoms
- Systemic embolization
- Enlarging valve vegetations with threatened embolization
- Heart rhythm and conduction disturbances
- Evidence of local extension of vegetation to surrounding myocardium

Surgical indications for patients with prosthetic valves include the above as well as:
- Fungal pathology
- Valve obstruction
- Unstable valve prosthesis
- New onset heart block
- Perivalvular leak

Patients treated with combined medical and surgical therapy have a greater survival rate than those treated with only medical therapy.

22. **What are the types of valve replacement?**

There are two major types of valve replacement: mechanical or bioprosthetic (tissue-type). There are advantages and disadvantages to both types of valves; therefore valve usage is patient-specific, and the type of valve used is determined by the discretion of the surgeon and/or patient preference (please refer to Chapter 16).

23. **Define prosthetic valve dysfunction or failure.**

A prosthetic valve has failed when it is necessary to undergo a repeat valve replacement. The most common causes of mechanical valve dysfunction are thromboembolism, bleeding, endocarditis, and thrombosis. Bioprosthetic valve dysfunction is usually caused by tissue deterioration. Bioprosthetic valve replacement typically occurs in approximately 25% of patients at 10-years postsurgery and 65% of patients at 15-years postsurgery. Patients under age 35 may have an accelerated rate of tissue deterioration.

24. **What is cardiac tamponade?**

Cardiac tamponade is the accumulation of fluid in the pericardium in an amount sufficient to cause serious obstruction to the inflow of blood to the ventricles.

This complication of cardiac surgery can be fatal without rapid diagnosis and treatment. This is usually seen in patients who have significant bleeding or have bleeding that has suddenly stopped.

25. What are the classic manifestations of cardiac tamponade?

The classic manifestations of cardiac tamponade are:
- Elevation and/or equilibrium of intracardiac pressures
- Restriction of ventricular filling
- Reduction of cardiac output
- Hypotension
- Widening mediastinum on chest x-ray
- Tachycardia
- Dysrhythmias

The quantity of fluid necessary to produce this critical state is variable. The fluid collection may be as little as 200 ml when the fluid develops rapidly or more than 2000 ml in slowly developing effusions where the pericardium has had the opportunity to stretch and adapt to an increasing volume. The diagnosis of cardiac tamponade is established by echocardiography. An echocardiogram is the gold standard for diagnosis; it allows us to differentiate between ventricular failure and tamponade.

26. How is cardiac tamponade treated?

The presence of cardiac tamponade or uncontrolled mediastinal bleeding requires immediate mediastinal exploration with identification and repair of the bleeding source. Evacuation of the blood collection usually produces immediate reversal of symptoms. Fluid resuscitation and blood transfusion are usually warranted as determined by the amount of blood loss. It is important that patent chest tubes are placed during chest evacuation to prevent further fluid collections. Correction of abnormal coagulation studies is imperative to prevent reoccurrence of tamponade.

27. What is the procedure for emergency mediastinal reexploration?

- Remove the sternal dressing.
- Pour antiseptic over chest area on skin.
- Place four sterile towels around the sternal incision.
- Open wound down to the sternum with knife.
- Cut sternal wires with a wire cutter or untwist ties.
- Use sternal retractor to expose the heart.
- Continue resuscitation with fluid and blood products.
- Place finger over bleeding site and suction excess blood from chest.
- Control and repair bleeding sites.
- Irrigate mediastinum with warm saline or antibiotic solution if available.
- Close chest incision.

28. What is multiple system organ failure following cardiac surgery?

Multiple system organ failure is a syndrome that describes patients who have failure of two or more organ systems. This is usually associated with a high death rate. The presumed cause of this syndrome in a postoperative cardiac surgery patient is a low cardiac output state and/or sepsis. The common organ systems that are affected are cardiac, respiratory, gastrointestinal, renal, and hepatic. Individually, failure of these organ systems can be devastating, but in combination the death rate increases with the number of involved organ systems. It is estimated that multiple system organ failure affects approximately 1% to 2% of postoperative cardiac surgery patients.

29. What is the incidence and treatment of postoperative sternal wound infections?

Sternal wound infections occur in approximately 2% of cardiac surgery procedures with a median sternotomy incision. These infections usually present about 10 days after the surgical procedure. Treatment includes antibiotic therapy, mediastinal reexploration, and sternal debridement with possible placement of muscle flaps.

30. What are the risk factors for development of postoperative sternal wound infections?

- Diabetes mellitus
- Obesity
- Chronic obstructive pulmonary disease
- Prolonged ventilatory support
- Bilateral internal mammary artery (IMA) usage
- Excessive mediastinal bleeding or multiple transfusions
- Impaired nutritional status
- Advanced age
- Low cardiac output syndromes requiring inotropic support
- Reoperations
- Prolonged cardiopulmonary bypass or surgical duration

31. What are the common anticoagulants used following cardiac surgery and what are their complications?

The most common anticoagulants used following cardiac surgery are heparin and warfarin (Coumadin). Most patients receive intravenous heparin following normalization of coagulation studies and cessation of operative bleeding. Warfarin therapy begins once the patient is stable and able to swallow. Heparin therapy continues until the warfarin levels, as measured by prothrombin time/INR, are at the suggested level for the underlying pathology being treated. Complications may arise because of these anticoagulants. The most prevalent complication is bleeding or hemorrhage. Other complications may include thrombocytopenia, thrombosis or embolus related to subtherapeutic anticoagulation, and anemia.

32. What gastrointestinal complications are common after cardiac surgery?

Gastrointestinal complications occur in about 1% to 2% of patients undergoing cardiac surgery. Causes of gastrointestinal complications may include paralytic ileus, cholecystitis, pancreatitis, gastrointestinal bleeding, mesenteric ischemia, diarrhea, and hepatic dysfunction.

33. How is rejection identified after heart transplantation?

Identification of organ rejection is most likely recognized during routine endomyocardial biopsies, which are performed regularly following transplant. Clinical signs of acute rejection may include bradyarrhythmias and low output syndrome. Diagnosis of organ rejection can only be confirmed by endomyocardial biopsy. Treatment of rejection is individualized to the patient; however, it will usually include high-dose corticosteroids and modification of immunosuppressive drugs.

34. What types of arrhythmia complications occur after cardiac surgery?

The most common postoperative arrhythmia is atrial tachyarrhythmia or atrial fibrillation. Approximately 11% to 40% of patients will develop atrial arrhythmias. The peak incidence of atrial arrhythmias occurs on postoperative days 2 and 3. Other arrhythmias noted in cardiac surgical patients can include ventricular arrhythmias (0.41% to 1.4% incidence) and bradyarrhythmias (0.8% to 3.4% incidence). Risk factors for increased incidence of cardiac arrhythmias include: history of arrhythmia, advanced age, type of surgery (valve surgery presents a higher risk than coronary revascularization), history of left ventricular dysfunction, hypertension, increased cardiopulmonary bypass time, hypomagnesemia, and inflammation caused by pericarditis.

35. What is the purpose of placement of temporary epicardial pacing wires after cardiac surgery?

Patients usually have two ventricular and two atrial pacemaker leads placed in their heart during an open-heart surgical procedure. These leads can be used for both diagnosis and treatment purposes. Diagnostically we can use the atrial pacemaker leads to distinguish atrial arrhythmias from their more dangerous ventricular arrhythmias. This is done by attaching the arm limb leads to the atrial wires on an electrocardiogram monitor. This will show atrial activity, therefore assisting with diagnosis of atrial arrhythmias. Temporary pacemaker leads are also used for treatment. We use a pacemaker to increase the heart rate to optimize hemodynamics in the postoperative period. We can also use atrial pacemaker wires to terminate reentrant atrial arrhythmias by rapid atrial pacing in select patients.

36. What does the pacemaker nomenclature represent?

Pacemaker settings usually have three capitalized letters representing the mode or type of pacing. The first letter represents the heart chamber that you are pacing, the second letter represents the heart chamber that the pacemaker is sensing, and the third letter represents the device's response to the impulses received. For example, VVI sensing would mean that we are pacing the ventricle, sensing the ventricle, and inhibiting pacing with intrinsic conduction.

37. **What is the infection risk of temporary pacing wires and how do we prevent it?**

Although the rate of sternal infections is low overall, it carries a high morbidity and mortality rate. It is possible that improper care of epicardial pacemaker wires could significantly increase the risk of developing a sternal infection. Nursing care of epicardial pacemaker sites should include daily dressing changes with or without antimicrobial ointment and aseptic cleansing of the site with povidone-iodine; of course, hand-washing before and after any contact with the patient is extremely important. Epicardial site care may vary with the institution.

38. **What is the most dreaded complication after temporary pacer wire removal?**

Cardiac tamponade. The procedure for removing pacer wires varies with the institution, but generally the patient is maintained on bed rest for 1 hour, and a chest x-ray and electrocardiogram are ordered. It is very important that the patient has adequate hemostasis before pacer wire removal.

Key Points

- Low cardiac output may be managed with inotropic medications, volume regulation, intraaortic balloon pumps, and ventricular assist devices.
- Endocarditis may occur at any time after cardiac valve surgery.
- Many factors may contribute to the development of sternal wound infections, such as diabetes mellitus, prolonged ventilation, steroid use preoperatively, use of internal thoracic arteries, and obesity.

Internet Resources

American College of Surgeons: College Guidelines:
http://www.facs.org/fellows_info/guidelines/cardiac.html

Looksmart: Cardiac Management in the ICU:
http://articles.findarticles.com/p/articles/mi_m0984/is_5_115/ai_54776356

BIBLIOGRAPHY

Alspach J, editor: *Core curriculum for critical care nursing*, Philadelphia, 1998, WB Saunders.

Baue, AE: Multiple organ failure, multiple organ dysfunction syndrome, and systemic inflammatory response syndrome. Why no magic bullets, *Arch Surg* 132(7):703-707, 1997.

Beery TA, Baas LS, Hichek CS: Infection precautions with temporary pacing leads: a descriptive study, *Heart Lung* 25(3):182-189, 1996.

Birjiniuk V: Patient outcomes in the assessment of myocardial injury following cardiac surgery, *Ann Thoracic Surg* 72(6):S2208-2212, 2001.

Bojar R: *Manual of Perioperative Care in Cardiac Surgery*, ed 3, Malden, Mass, 1999, Blackwell Science.

Braunwald E, Fauci AS, Kasper DL, Hauser SL, Longo DL, Jameson JL: *Harrison's Principals of Internal Medicine*, ed 15, New York, 2003, McGraw-Hill.

Christensen DM: The ventricular assist device: an overview, *Acute Care Cardiol* 35(4):945-959, 2000.

Chung MK: Cardiac surgery: postoperative arrhythmias, *Crit Care Med* 28(10)(suppl):N136-N144, 2000.

El Gamel A, Deiraniya AK, Rahman AN, Campbell CS, Yonan NA: Orthotopic heart transplantation: does atrial preservation improve cardiac output after transplantation, *J Heart Lung Transplant* 12:564-571, 1996.

Gill R, Murkin JM: Neuropsychologic dysfunction after cardiac surgery; what is the problem, *J Cardiothor Vasc Anesthesia* 112:1036-1045, 1996.

Higgins TL, Yared JP, Ryan T: Immediate postoperative care of cardiac surgical patients, *J Cardiothor Vasc Anesthesia* 10:643-658, 1996.

Hirsh J, Dalen JE, Deykin D, Poller L, Bussey H: Oral anticoagulants. Mechanism of action, clinical effectiveness, and optimal therapeutic range, *Chest* 108(suppl):231S-246S, 1995.

Lay TD, Puntillo KA, Miaskowski CA, Wallhagen MI: Analgesics prescribed and administered in intensive care cardiac surgery patients: does patient age make a difference, *Prog Cardiovasc Nurs* 11(4):17-24, 1996.

Ley S: The Thoratec ventricular assist device: Nursing guidelines, *AACN Clin Iss Crit Care Nurs* 2:529-544, 1999.

McKhann GM, Goldsborough MA, Borowicz LM, Mellits ED, Brookmeyer R, Quaskey SA, Baumgartner WA, Cameron DE, Stuart RS, Gardner TJ: Predictors of stroke risk in coronary artery bypass patients, *Ann Thoracic Surg* 63:516-521, 1997.

Niederhauser U, Vogt M, Vogt P, Genoni M, Kunzli A, Turina MI: Cardiac surgery in a high-risk group of patients: is prolonged postoperative antibiotic prophylaxis effective, *J Thoracic Cardiovasc Surg* 114:162-168, 1997.

Nielsen D, Sellgren J, Ricksten SE: Quality of life after cardiac surgery complicated by multiple organ failure, *Crit Care Med* 25(1):52-57, 1997.

Ommen SR, Odell JA, Stanton MS: Current concepts: atrial arrhythmias after cardiothoracic surgery, *N Engl J Med* 336(20):1429-1434, 1997.

Robollo MH, Bernal JM, Llorca J, Rabasa JM, Revuelta JM: Nosocomial infections in patients having cardiovascular operations; a multivariate analysis of risk factors, *J Thoracic Cardiovasc Surg* 112:908-913, 1996.

Shorten GD, Comunale ME: Heparin-induced thrombocytopenia, *J Cardiothor Vasc Anesthesia* 10:521-530, 1996.

Torchiana DF, Hirsch G, Buckley MJ, et al: Intraaortic balloon pumping for cardiac support: trends in practice and outcome, 1968 to 1995, *J Thoracic Cardiovasc Surg* 113:758-769, 1997.

Tsang J, Brush B: Patient-controlled analgesia in postoperative cardiac surgery, *Anaesthesia Intensive Care* 27(5):464-470, 1999.

Vlessis AA, Hovaguimiam H, Jaggers J, Ahmad A, Starr A: Infective endocarditis: ten-year review of medical and surgical therapy, *Ann Thoracic Surg* 61:1217-1222, 1996.

Vlessis AA, Khaki A, Grunkemeier GL, Li HH, Star A: Risk, diagnosis, and management of prosthetic valve endocarditis: a review, *J Heart Valve Disord* 6:443-465, 1997.

Emergent Bedside Sternotomy

Gerald T. Rankin and Kathleen Shaughnessy

1. What is an emergent bedside sternotomy?

It is a potentially life-saving surgical procedure intended to restore hemody-namic stability to a postoperative cardiac patient. For an experienced surgeon, the presence of an existing median sternotomy allows rapid reopening and visualization of the mediastinum, and prompt initiation of life-saving inter-ventions. This life-saving procedure is performed in an ICU setting in the early postoperative period and is therefore referred to as an emergent bedside sternotomy (EBS).

2. What is a median sternotomy?

A median sternotomy is a vertical midline incision extending from below the suprasternal notch to a point just distal to the xyphoid process. The length of the incision is dependent on surgeon preference. Median sternotomy is the traditional incision used for cardiac surgery as this approach allows for optimal visualization of the heart and mediastinum.

3. Who typically has the responsibility of recognizing the potential need for an EBS?

The postoperative management of the cardiac surgery patient is a team effort. The team typically consists of the surgeon, anesthesiologist, cardiologist, pul-monologist, certified registered nurse practitioner (CRNP) or physician assis-tant (PA), and bedside registered nurse (RN). While all disciplines are important it is imperative that the bedside RN recognizes the potential for an EBS and communicates promptly and frequently to the appropriate team members. The RN is typically the only team member that monitors the patient around the clock and therefore plays a major role in the recognition of the potential need for an EBS.

4. **What is the primary goal of the RN in the care of a hemodynamically unstable postoperative cardiac surgery patient?**

The primary goal of the RN is to restore hemodynamic stability and avoid the need for an EBS. If reexploration of the mediastinum is necessary, it is preferable in most institutions to return the patient to the sterile operating room environment. Therefore the RN needs to recognize the potential for reexploration, frequently communicate with appropriate team members, and keep the patient stable enough to return to the operating room in a controlled manner. If an EBS is necessary, the RN needs to continue efforts to maintain hemodynamic stability until preparation for the procedure can be accomplished. A combination of blood volume resuscitation, pharmacological inotropic support, ACLS protocol, and assurance of chest tube patency is typically needed to maintain a relative level of hemodynamic stability.

5. **How often is surgical reexploration needed in the immediate postoperative period of cardiac surgery?**

Approximately 3% to 7% of postoperative cardiac surgery patients require surgical reexploration. Patients who have undergone prolonged cardiopulmonary bypass (>120 minutes), cardiac reoperations, or valvular repair/replacements tend to demonstrate a greater likelihood of postoperative surgical reexploration.

6. **Name three primary life-threatening complications that would necessitate initiation of an EBS.**

- Cardiac tamponade
- Excessive mediastinal bleeding
- Refractory lethal dysrhythmias

7. **What is cardiac tamponade?**

Cardiac tamponade is a collection of fluid in the posterior pericardial sac or mediastinal space that compromises right ventricular filling. The fluid accumulation around the heart does not allow for normal relaxation during diastole. This impaired relaxation results in reduced cardiac filling and therefore cardiac output. Acute life-threatening situations occur because of the rate of fluid accumulation rather than the volume of accumulation. The pericardium can accommodate 1 to 2 liters of fluid before cardiac deterioration occurs if the accumulation is gradual. Rapid fluid accumulation can cause tamponade with as little as 100 ml of fluid. In the postoperative cardiac surgery patient, this fluid is most often blood or clots not adequately drained by mediastinal chest tubes.

8. **What are the clinical signs of cardiac tamponade?**

Signs of cardiac tamponade	
Early Signs	**Late Signs**
Rising CVP (except in hypovolemic patient)	Low cardiac index
Tachycardia	Hypotension
Tachypnea	Distant heart sounds
Jugular vein distention	Equalization of CVP and PAD
Anxiety	Widening mediastinum on chest x-ray
Poor peripheral pulses	ECG disturbances (bradycardia, cardiac arrest)
Cessation of chest tube drainage	Low voltage on ECG
Decrease in urinary output	Pulsus paradoxus
	RV collapse on echocardiography

9. **Are there classic signs of cardiac tamponade?**

    Cardiac tamponade should be suspected when atrial pressures are increasing with the concurrent onset of hypotension and distant heart sounds. This triad of signs—*Beck's triad*—are often referred to as classical signs of cardiac tamponade. It is important to understand that all patients do not demonstrate the complete triad.

10. **What patients are at risk for cardiac tamponade?**

    * Patients with a history of bleeding diatheses
    * Patients that have undergone repeat sternotomy procedures
    * Patients with recent epicardial pacing wire removal
    * Patients on anticoagulation therapy preoperatively

11. **Do all patients who develop cardiac tamponade require an EBS?**

    No. All patients in cardiac tamponade do not need surgical reexploration. Early recognition of tamponade symptoms and aggressive management of volume resuscitation efforts may allow hemodynamic stability and ensure safe return to the operating room. Diagnosed in its late stage, cardiac tamponade will most likely result in an EBS because of the high likelihood of life-threatening hemodynamic instability.

12. **What are the two primary causes for excessive mediastinal bleeding?**

    * Medical bleeding
    * Surgical bleeding

13. What is medical bleeding?

Medical bleeding is bleeding secondary to the abnormalities of coagulation. The etiology of coagulopathy is often multifactorial. Preoperative use of Coumadin, aspirin, heparin, NSAIDs, GPIIb/IIIa antagonists (ReoPro, Aggrastat), fibrinolytic drugs (tissue plasminogen activator, streptokinase, urokinase), and antiplatelet medications (Plavix) increases the risk for coagulopathies to occur. Metabolic disorders such as uremia and liver dysfunction predispose patients to possible coagulopathies. Inadequate patient rewarming, inadequate reversal of heparin at the conclusion of cardiopulmonary bypass (CPB), and alterations in the coagulation cascade in addition to platelet destruction and dysfunction secondary to CPB are significant factors in postoperative bleeding. Employment of an intraaortic balloon pump (IABP) or ventricular assist device (VAD) alters platelet function and can contribute to abnormalities of coagulation.

14. What is excessive mediastinal bleeding?

There is no definitive answer to this frequently asked question. Clinical judgment and experience are important components in ultimately defining excessive bleeding. Any amount of bleeding that leads to hemodynamic collapse is excessive, and immediate intervention is required. Acute onset of massive bleeding (for example, 500- to 1000-ml chest tube output in 15 minutes) or bleeding that persists despite normalization of coagulation parameters is excessive bleeding. As a general rule, chest tube output that exceeds 500 ml/hour in the first hour postoperatively, 400 ml/hour during the first 2 hours, 300 ml/hour during the first 3 hours, and 200 ml/hour during the first 4 to 6 hours can be used as a guideline for excessive bleeding.

15. Do all patients experiencing excessive bleeding require an EBS?

No. Excessive bleeding that does not taper, despite correction of suspected coagulopathy, will require surgical reexploration. In most institutions surgical reexploration is preferred in a controlled operating room environment. If the patient is massively bleeding, an EBS is likely because hemodynamic collapse nearly always accompanies massive bleeding.

16. What are the complications associated with an EBS?

The complications associated with EBS include increased risk of mediastinitis or sternal nonunion, anoxic encephalopathy, prolonged mechanical ventilatory support, or perforation of a patent LIMA/RIMA graft.

17. How is internal cardiac massage/internal defibrillation used during EBS?

Once the sternotomy is performed, the surgeon or surgical designee ceases to perform external compressions and internal cardiac massage begins. Internal cardiac massage ensures continued limited blood volume circulation. Internal defibrillation at 10 to 20 joules may be attempted to terminate ventricular tachycardia or fibrillation.

18. **What emergency equipment is needed during the EBS?**
    - Code cart
    - Sterile internal defibrillator pads
    - Sternotomy cart, including:
       - scalpel, knife handler, wire cutters, and sternal retractors
       - sterile drapes and towels
       - Yankauer suction tip, suction tubing, and canisters
       - forceps, needle holders, suture materials, pledgets, sterile lap sponges
       - sternal wires, bone wax, and needle counter

19. **Describe the EBS procedure and the roles of the team members.**

    The tamponade or excessive bleeding situation is identified and reported by the bedside RN to the surgeon or his/her designee. The decision is then made to proceed with EBS. The RN notifies the anesthesiologist/anesthetist, respiratory therapist, attending cardiologist, covering intensivist/resident/PA/NP of the anticipated procedure. The anesthesiologist/anesthetist may need to intubate the patient (if not already done) and coordinate medication administration. Blood products are obtained and administered by additional nursing staff. Dressings are removed from the patient's chest, and the area is prepped with Betadine. Everyone in the patient's room must wear a surgical mask and hat. The surgeon and assistant don sterile gowns and gloves. Sometimes the cardiac operating room staff may be available to assist the surgeon. The sternotomy kit is opened on a bedside table while sterile drapes are placed on the patient. Staff is kept to a minimum to reduce risk of infection to the patient. Suction and tubing are attached to wall suction systems, and additional chest tube drainage systems are available. The RN coordinates room activity and ensures needed items are available from the pharmacy and store room. Additional antibiotics may be administered because of the lack of a sterile environment due to the emergent nature of the situation. The bleeding sites are often identified and repaired at the bedside. Once the bleeding is corrected, the patient's sternum is rewired and their skin is closed.

 Key Points

- The staff nurse has a vital role in the resuscitation of the patient after an emergent bedside sternotomy.
- Indications for emergency sternotomy include tamponade, excessive bleeding, and refractory arrhythmias.
- Patients on Plavix before surgery are at risk for increased bleeding postoperatively.

Internet Resources

LookSmart: Unexpected Cardiac Arrest after Cardiac Surgery:
http://www.findarticles.com/p/articles/mi_m0984/is_n1_v1113/ai_20369758

Emedicine Article on Cardiac Tamponade:
http://www.emedicine.com/med/topic283.htm

BIBLIOGRAPHY

Bojar R: *Manual of Perioperative Care in Cardiac Surgery*, ed 3, Malden, Mass, 1999, Blackwell Science.

Finkelmeier BA: *Cardiothoracic Surgical Nursing*, ed 2, Philadelphia, 2000, JB Lippincott.

Section II

Thoracic

Pulmonary Disorders

Anne Marie Kuzma and Karen Steinke

1. What is bronchiectasis?

Bronchiectasis is a disease of the airways that causes permanently dilated bronchi, usually in the proximal airways. Bronchiectasis is subdivided into two types: wet and dry. Wet bronchiectasis refers to airways that are inflamed and edematous and full of purulent sputum. A patient with wet bronchiectasis produces a large amount of mucus on a regular basis. With dry bronchiectasis the affected airways are ulcerated with mucosal erosion and may develop abscesses. Bronchiectasis may be focal or diffuse, and in almost one third of all cases it is bilateral. Focal bronchiectasis is often the result of foreign body aspiration or adenopathy, and benign tumors.

2. Which pulmonary functions are altered with the diagnosis of bronchiectasis?

Pulmonary function tests show a reduction in airflow rates, forced vital capacity (FVC), and forced expiratory volume in 1 second (FEV_1). As the disease becomes advanced, hypoxemia is also present.

3. What are some of the common illnesses that may lead to bronchiectasis?

This disease of the airways is caused by bronchial wall destruction because of infection, inhalation of noxious chemicals, immunological reactions, or vascular abnormalities.

4. What are the typical signs and symptoms associated with bronchiectasis?

Severe pneumonia with lingering symptoms, a persistent residual cough, and dyspnea are common symptoms associated with bronchiectasis although occasionally a patient has no symptoms. Symptoms are insidious; they usually appear after a respiratory infection and gradually worsen over a period of years. As the disease progresses, the cough usually becomes productive; there also may be wheezing and shortness of breath (SOB) on exertion. Physical findings are nonspecific: crackles over the affected lung, decreased breath sounds, and prolonged expiration or wheezing.

5. How is the diagnosis of bronchiectasis confirmed?

Bronchiectasis is suspected in anyone with persistent cough, progressive short-ness of breath, and wheezing after a respiratory infection. A chest x-ray may show hyperinflation and/or increased vascular markings from peribronchial fibrosis and intrabronchial secretions. Characteristics seen on a high-resolution CAT scan (HRCT) are dilated airways (tram lines); tram lines have a signet ring appearance with a luminal diameter almost twice the size of the adjacent vessel. Associated conditions need to be investigated, particularly cystic fibrosis, immune deficiencies, and any predisposing congenital abnormalities.

6. Describe the treatment of bronchiectasis.

Treatment is directed against infections, secretions, and airway obstruction. A sputum culture and sensitivity is needed to target the appropriate antibiotic(s). The choice of agents depends on the result of the sputum culture for aerobes, anaerobes, and mycobacteria. Sputum cultures usually will contain both gram-positive and gram-negative organisms. *Haemophilus influenza* and *Staphylococcus aureus* are the two most common microorganisms. Broad-spectrum antibiotics (ampicillin or amoxicillin, Bactrim, macrolides, or a second-generation cephalosporin) are often the drugs of choice. Antibiotics should be repeated at the first sign of recurring infection: increase in purulence and quantity of spu-tum. If infections reoccur often, then a prolonged course of antibiotics may be required. The duration may be 14 to 21 days. Whether prophylactic antibiotics reduce the frequencies of recurrent infections is controversial. Suppressive antibiotics are thought to reduce the amount of bacteria, but there is no defini-tive answer if long-term continuous therapy is better than intermittent therapy. The goal is to prevent development of resistant organisms such as *Pseudomonas*. An example of an oral regimen is antibiotic use 7 to 10 days each month. Another regimen is to use an antibiotic for 3 to 6 months. A fluroquinolone such as ciprofloxacin 500 to 750 mg every 12 hours may be effective for a long period of time. If resistance to oral medications becomes problematic, a course of aerosol or intravenous antibiotics may be necessary. As the disease progresses and the microorganisms become resistant to oral antibiotics, a semipermanent intravenous access may need to be inserted.

Complications must be managed as well. Patients need to be monitored for the development of hypoxemia, hemoptysis, and respiratory failure (cor pul-monale). Bronchodilators, theophylline, and corticosteroids can be used to treat airflow hyperreactivity, assist sputum clearance, and reduce inflammation. Chronic hypoxemia should be treated with oxygen. Supplemental oxygen should be prescribed if the PaO_2 is <55 mm Hg on room air or if the SaO_2 falls below 87% on room air. Oxygen therapy may also be recommended if the patient has secondary pulmonary hypertension. Massive hempotysis may require endo-bronchial balloon tamponade or selective embolization. Patients with bronchiectasis should avoid inhaling cigarette smoke or other lung irritants and also refrain from taking sedatives and antitussives.

Certain procedures may be helpful for patients during an acute flare. Postural drainage, including clapping and vibration, can be performed twice a day to help loosen secretions. There are several newer devices that can be used in conjunction with chest physical therapy. Theravest, an electrical device that vibrates the chest wall and helps mobilize secretions, and Flutter Valve, a hand-held device that contains a ball bearing that transmits vibrating waves back to the airways, are now frequently prescribed for both home and hospital use.

Nebulized medications such as Pulmozyme break down the DNA in purulent sputum and may benefit select patients with bronchiectasis.

7. What is the most common cause of community-acquired pneumonia?

The organism responsible for approximately 50% of acute community-acquired pneumonia cases is *Streptococcus pneumoniae.* In the elderly, community-acquired pneumonia is frequently caused by aerobic gram-negative bacilli as well as by *Staphylococcus aureus.* This may be attributable to increased colonization of the pharynx by gram-negative rods secondary to a serious underlying disease, prior antibiotic therapy, and a decrease in overall physical activity. During winter months the elderly are at risk for influenza pneumonia. The clinical presentation of community-acquired pneumonia varies with the cause and the comorbidities of the person affected.

8. Describe the clinical course associated with pneumonia.

Pneumonia resulting from pyogenic organisms such as *Streptococcal pneumoniae, Staphylococcus aureus,* or *Hemophilus influenzae* usually presents with a fever, productive cough, chest pain, and shortness of breath. The respiratory rate is increased, and the patient may need to use accessory muscles. The clinical picture will vary depending on the age of the patient, the immune state, and the type of microorganism. The patient with bacterial pneumonia manifests respiratory distress and often needs to be observed in an intensive care unit. Physical examination of the affected lung shows evidence of consolidation, increased vocal fremitus, and dullness to percussion, crackles, whispered pectoriloquy, and egophony.

9. What is the incidence of pneumonia-associated mortality?

An estimated 50,000 patients will die from pneumonia annually. About 5% of all patients who develop pneumonia will expire. If bacteremia is also present the rate increases to 20%.

10. What are the risk factors associated with mortality in the patient with pneumonia?

Advanced age and underlying medical conditions such as previous splenectomy, cirrhosis, chronic obstructive lung disease (COPD), immunodeficiency syndromes, and malignancies are strongly associated with increased mortality.

If leukopenia, jaundice, extrapulmonary complications, and involvement of three or more lobes of the lung occur, the prognosis is poor.

11. **What is the most common type of community-acquired pneumonia?**

Pneumococcal pneumonia.

12. **What diagnostic tests are usually ordered in a patient with suspected pneumonia?**

- Chest radiograph
- Sputum cultures
- Blood cultures
- Complete blood count

13. **What is the frequency of nosocomial pneumonia?**

Nosocomial pneumonia is the second leading hospital-acquired infection. Nearly 1% of patients admitted to the hospital develop pneumonia. About one third of these patients will die. Sixty percent of ICU patients will develop pneumonia. The most common microorganisms are gram-negative bacilli and *Staphylococcus aureus*. The microorganism responsible for nosocomial pneumonia infections will vary between institutions.

14. **What hospital variables may predispose patients to pneumonia?**

- Aspiration
- Mechanical ventilation
- Feeding tubes
- Sedation
- Colonization of the gastrointestinal tract, which may be associated with decreased gastric acidity from the use of histamine blockers

15. **Should empirical antibiotics be used in the prevention of nosocomial pneumonia?**

Because of the high mortality associated with nosocomial pneumonia and the presence of resistant organisms in most hospitals, the use of broad-spectrum antibiotics is begun as soon as pneumonia is suspected. Once an organism is identified, the antibiotic can be targeted toward the pathogen. Patients who have been hospitalized for greater than 3 days and are seriously ill are likely to be colonized with resistant gram-negative organisms.

16. **What are the most frequent microorganisms seen in patients on mechanical ventilation?**

Pseudomonas and *Enterobacter* species are frequent organisms in patients on mechanical ventilation.

17. What are some of the clinical signs associated with atypical pneumonia?

- Low-grade fever
- Nonproductive cough
- Myalgia

18. What are the common causes of atypical pneumonia?

- *Mycoplasma*
- Viruses
- *Chlamydia*

19. What is a solitary pulmonary nodule (SPN)?

A SPN is a radiographic finding of a small ($\leq$4 cm) round density surrounded by normal lung tissue without intrathoracic adenopathy or associated atelectasis. The nodule may be calcified or noncalcified; the border may be irregular or sharp.

20. What are the causes of SPNs?

The most common cause of a SPN is granuloma. These may be a result of prior lung infections, such as histoplasmosis and tuberculosis. Neoplasms are bronchogenic or carcinogenic, or they metastasize from extrathoracic malignancies. Bronchogenic carcinoma accounts for an estimated one third of all SPNs.

21. How is a solitary pulmonary nodule diagnosed?

- Physical examination
- Induced sputum with hypertonic saline
- Chest CT scan
- Biopsy

22. Define chronic obstructive pulmonary disease (COPD).

COPD is a disease characterized by airflow limitations. The disease states include emphysema and chronic bronchitis.

23. What is the prevalence of COPD?

Approximately 14 million people in the United States have COPD. Emphysema is the fourth leading cause of death in the United States.

24. What is the correlation between cigarette smoking and chronic obstructive pulmonary disease (COPD)?

Cigarette smoking is the leading cause of emphysema. A total of 75 million U.S. citizens smoke. Cigarette smoking is thought to induce an imbalance between proteases and antiproteases in the lungs. This interaction increases elastase activity, causing destruction of the elastic fibers of the alveolar walls. The benefits of smoking cessation are well established. In younger smokers (<35 years) who have mild COPD, the FEV_1 will return to normal after the patient stops smoking. In older patients cessation of smoking will slow the progress of the disease but not eliminate the disease.

25. Describe the physiological effects of chronic obstructive pulmonary disease (COPD).

The excessive and tenacious secretions common in emphysema occlude airway lumens, limiting airflow. Contraction of smooth muscles in airways and bronchial wall edema and inflammation also decrease luminal diameters. As the lung's parenchyma is destroyed, the tethering forces exerted on the airway lumens are diminished. Moderate sized airways become floppy during forced expiration. Pulmonary mechanics, including expiratory flow rates and volumes, are diminished during the expiratory cycle, which prolongs expiration time and prevents complete emptying of the affected alveoli. The increased lung volumes flatten the diaphragm. Therefore in patients with COPD the work of breathing is increased because of the increase in airway resistance and the altered respiratory muscle mechanics. Patients with COPD usually seek medical attention for treatment of a respiratory infection or when their shortness of breath interferes with their activities.

26. What are the two classifications of patients with COPD?

• Pink puffer
• Blue bloater

27. Describe the difference between the pink puffer and the blue bloater.

A pink puffer is tachypneic with labored repetitions and pursed lip breathing. Arterial oxygenation is usually preserved. A blue bloater is a patient who appears chronically cyanotic (arterial hypoxemia) and may exhibit hypercapnia, leg edema, and right-sided heart failure. Patients tend to be obese, and often produce mucus on a regular basis. This classification of COPD patients is used to define the underlying process. The blue bloater is associated with chronic bronchitis, and the pink puffer is associated with emphysema. This classification has become less useful because there is a significant amount of overlap and few patients fall exclusively into either subset.

28. What are the common physical examination findings in patients with COPD?

• Diminished breath sounds
• Expiratory wheezing
• Prolonged expiratory phase
• Increased anterior-posterior diameter of the chest

- Limited excursion of the diaphragm
- Signs of right-sided heart failure, if the patient is hypoxemic

29. **Describe the treatment protocol for a patient admitted with acute exacerbation of chronic obstructive pulmonary disease (COPD).**

Patients admitted with shortness of breath related to emphysema need to be monitored for respiratory failure. Hospitalized patients should be switched from meter-dosed inhalers to the nebulized route. Bronchodilator dosage needs to be intensified during exacerbation. Nebulized treatments of albuterol, a short-acting bronchodilator, are increased to 5.0 to 7.5 mg every 2 to 3 hours. Treatments of Ipratropium bromide, an anticholinergic agent that decreases vagal tone, inhibits smooth muscle contraction, and decreases secretions, should be administered every 6 hours. It is important to ensure that all bronchodilators are given as prescribed to prevent excessive hyperinflation.

Theophylline may be used chronically or started during an exacerbation. The mechanism in which theophylline works is unknown, but this agent decreases dyspnea and airway obstruction. Optimal bronchodilator effects may occur in the low therapeutic range (5 to 15 mg/dl).

Pulse dose steroids are started in patients in exacerbation. As the patient's breathlessness improves, the steroid dose can be decreased and then tapered, as well as the bronchodilator dose.

Intubation should be avoided as much as possible. Noninvasive positive pressure ventilation can be used to decrease breathlessness, improve oxygenation, and lower carbon dioxide levels. Vapotherm, high-flow humidified oxygen, has been shown to decrease breathlessness during acute exacerbation.

30. **What is the natural progression of COPD?**

The natural progression of emphysema is often correlated to the forced expiratory volume in 1 second (FEV_1). Median survival is approximately 10 years when FEV_1 is 1.4 L, 4 years when FEV_1 is 1 L, and less then 2 years when FEV_1 is 0.5 L.

31. **What is tuberculosis?**

Tuberculosis (TB) refers to a disease caused by *Mycobacterium tuberculosis*. TB is a nonmotile bacillus. TB is a major world health problem with an estimated 8 million new cases and about 3 million deaths each year.

32. **Which populations have the highest incidence of tuberculosis?**

The disease is most prevalent in urban areas. Several populations have been identified as having a high incidence of TB. These groups include:
- Prison inmates
- Alcoholics
- Drug-dependent persons
- Homeless persons

- HIV-infected persons
- Persons in residential care facilities

33. How is tuberculosis transmitted?

Infection occurs primarily by inhalation of respiratory droplets aerosolized by coughing, sneezing, or talking. Initial infection usually occurs in the lower lung fields because of the greater distribution of ventilation to the lung bases. Bacterial multiplication proceeds slowly, both in the initial focus and in metastatic foci. Approximately 6 to 8 weeks after initial infection, specific cell-mediated immunity develops, providing effective killing of most organisms and containment of infection by the formation of granulomas. The TB skin test becomes positive at this time. Reactivation infection occurs in about 10% of infected patients. Reactivation occurs within 2 years after initial infection. When reactivation occurs it is most common in the apical posterior segment of the upper lobes of the lungs, which are rarely the site of primary infection. Primary infection is usually asymptomatic.

34. What are the common manifestations associated with tuberculosis?

- Anorexia
- Weight loss
- Fever
- Night sweats
- Hemoptysis

35. How is tuberculosis treated?

Multiple drugs should be used to prevent the emergence of drug-resistant organisms. If treatment failures occur, drugs need to be changed in combination rather than singularly. Single daily drug doses are preferred, and sputum cultures for acid-fast bacilli (AFB) should be repeated. No matter what regimen is chosen, it is important to follow patients closely to ensure compliance and to monitor drug effectiveness and toxicity. Monthly liver function studies should be performed because of the hepatic toxicity associated with some of the medications.

36. What is a pleural effusion?

A pleural effusion is an accumulation of free fluid within the pleural space.

37. Describe the fluid characteristics of a pleural effusion.

The accumulated fluid in a pleural effusion is referred to as transudate or exudate. A transudative fluid occurs when fluid is allowed to cross from the capillary bed into the pleural space as a result of an increase in hydrostatic pressure. This fluid is clear and straw-colored in appearance. It has a low concentration of protein and blood cells. An exudative fluid occurs when the formation and absorption of pleural fluid are altered. This frequently occurs secondary to an infection. An exudate fluid may appear turbid, cloudy, or blood-tinged and have both protein and L-lactate dehydrogenase (LDH) present on laboratory analysis.

38. What causes a pleural effusion?

Transudative effusions are commonly caused by conditions such as congestive heart failure, ascites, cirrhosis, peritoneal dialysis, and pulmonary embolism. Exudative effusions may result from tuberculosis, empyema, parapneumonic processes, cancer, trauma, collagen disorders, and pancreatitis.

39. What are the signs and symptoms associated with a pleural effusion?

Most often the symptoms accompanying a pleural effusion are associated with the underlying cause of the effusion; that is, they relate to the size of the effusion and the rate of accumulation of fluid in the pleural space. Patients with an effusion less than 300 ml frequently do not have any symptoms, and the effusion may resolve spontaneously. With larger effusions, the patient may complain of dyspnea, pleuritic chest pain, tachycardia, cough, fever, chills, or hemoptysis. Auscultation of the lungs will reveal decreased breath sounds or a friction rub over the involved area.

40. Describe the chest x-ray findings associated with a pleural effusion.

The chest x-ray is the major diagnostic test used to identify a pleural effusion. Posteroanterior (PA) and lateral views will generally identify an effusion. With as little as 100 ml of pleural fluid, a blunting of the costophrenic angle can be seen on the lateral chest x-ray. Blunting will be seen on the PA view with 200 ml or more of pleural fluid. Identification of the underlying cause of the effusion is also necessary for effective treatment.

41. What is the role of thoracentesis in the management of a pleural effusion?

A thoracentesis is performed to achieve relief of symptoms by draining fluid from the pleural space. The patient should be placed in an upright position for this procedure, preferably resting their arms on a table while sitting on the edge of the bed. The fluid should be removed slowly with no more than 1000 to 1500 ml removed at a time. If the patient complains of chest pain or begins to cough, the procedure should be stopped. Additionally, the fluid obtained should be sent for laboratory examination. The presence of protein, LDH, red cells, or white cells would indicate that the effusion is an exudate. If the fluid appears cloudy or blood-tinged or has pus in it, a Gram stain should be done. A repeat chest x-ray is done after the procedure to ensure that a pneumothorax has not developed and to assess the effectiveness of the thoracentesis.

42. What is a chylothorax?

A chylothorax is a pleural effusion caused by the presence of chyle. Chyle is a milky fluid composed of lymphatic fluid and fat. This type of effusion is caused by either trauma to the lymphatic system or neoplastic disease. Chylothorax fluid may not always appear cloudy. If chyle or neoplasm is suspected, thoracentesis fluid should be sent for Gram stain and cytology.

43. What is an empyema?

An empyema is an exudative pleural effusion. There are three stages of development for an empyema: exudative stage, fibropurulent stage, and organizing stage. During this staging process, the empyema progresses from a sterile free-flowing fluid to a loculated infected site with lung entrapment.

44. How is an empyema diagnosed?

- Thoracentesis fluid that reveals either purulence or a positive Gram stain
- Chest CT scan

45. What are the most common bacterial organisms associated with an empyema?

The common causative organisms are *Staphylococcus, Haemophilus influenza, Escherichia coli,* and *Pseudomonas.*

46. Describe the treatment of an empyema.

Successful treatment of an empyema requires antibiotic therapy and drainage of the infected area. Typically, a chest tube is placed in the dependent area of the effusion. The tube may be connected to either water seal drainage or suction. If the patient fails to respond to this therapy, other interventions are necessary. The health care provider may inject a fibrinolytic agent such as urokinase or streptokinase, which breaks up the fibrin in the loculation and allows it to drain. A surgical alternative may include a decortication, which allows the surgeon to manually break up the areas of loculation and then place a chest tube. This allows for the free flow of infected fluid out of the loculated area.

47. What is a pulmonary embolus?

A pulmonary embolus (PE) occurs when a venous thrombus lodges in the vasculature of one of the lungs. A PE is not seen as an independent disease but is associated with another disease process.

48. What are the causes of a pulmonary embolus?

A PE can also occur as a result of other fluids/material that enter the vasculature. Deep vein thrombus, amniotic fluid during pregnancy, fat embolus, air, and iatrogenic causes are all sources of a pulmonary embolus.

49. **Who are the patients at risk for a pulmonary embolus from a deep vein thrombus?**

Three factors contribute to a patient's risk for developing a deep vein thrombus (DVT) and thus a PE. Venous stasis as associated with prolonged bed rest, hypercoagulability as seen in patients with disseminated intravascular coagulation, and vascular injury from trauma or surgery are referred to as Virchow's triad and can help identify patients at risk for the development of a DVT.

50. **What is the best therapy available in treating a PE?**

The very best treatment for a PE is prevention. Identification of the patients at risk and implementation of therapies directed at prevention of a DVT will do the most to prevent a PE from occurring. Early ambulation after surgery, the use of intermittent compression devices, and the use of prophylactic heparin or warfarin are common effective therapies.

51. **What are the signs and symptoms of a pulmonary embolus?**

The classic signs of a PE are actually rarely seen, because only a small percentage of patients actually present with these complaints. The signs and symptoms may include:
   - Dyspnea
   - Pleuritic chest pain
   - Hemoptysis
   - Cough
   - Splinting of the ribs with breathing
   - Tachycardia
   - Hypotension
   - Near syncope
   - Apprehension

52. **What diagnostic studies are used in identifying a pulmonary embolus?**

A chest x-ray, a ventilation/perfusion (VQ) scan of the lungs, a CT scan, and measurement of arterial blood gas are useful in the diagnosis of a PE. The gold standard is a pulmonary angiogram.

Chest x-ray is primarily used to exclude any other reasons for the patient's symptoms, such as a pneumothorax.

VQ scan is a nuclear medicine study that compares ventilation defects in the lungs with perfusion (vascular) defects. In the case of a pulmonary embolus, ventilation is usually normal but there is a defect in perfusion. If the VQ scan is negative then a PE is ruled out, but if the scan shows a low to high probability of a PE, then further testing is required to confirm a PE.

CT scan is capable of detecting defective filling in the segmental or larger pulmonary arteries but not in subsegmental arteries. Positive CT scan results in association with other signs and symptoms can help confirm the diagnosis of a PE. A negative CT scan does not rule out a PE especially if other clinical signs and symptoms support its presence.

Arterial blood gas measurements will show respiratory alkalosis and hypoxemia. However, the absence of hypoxemia does not rule out a PE.

53. Describe the treatment of a PE.

A PE is treated as an emergent situation. Treatment focuses on emergent relief of symptoms and identification of the underlying source of the PE. Anticoagulation should be started immediately. Typically, an infusion of heparin will be started. The purpose of this infusion is not to dissolve the clot but to prevent further thrombosis (inhibit growth of the PE). This allows the fibrinolytic system to proceed with the process of naturally dissolving the embolus. Low molecular weight dextran may be used as an alternative clot-preventing medication. For long-term anticoagulation, warfarin, aspirin, or other antiplatelet drugs are used.

54. What is the role of thrombolytic therapy in the treatment of a pulmonary embolus?

Thrombolytic therapy such as streptokinase, tissue plasminogen activator (TPA), or urokinase is typically used in the management of a pulmonary embolus that is causing hemodynamic instability or severe respiratory compromise.

55. What is sarcoidosis?

Sarcoidosis is a multisystem granulomatous disease with unknown etiology. Past studies suggest that the disease may be caused by environmental factors (exposure to the metal beryllium) or infectious agents *(Mycobacterium tuberculosis)*; it has also been suggested that there may be an inherited genetic component. None of these theories have been conclusively proven.

56. Describe the epidemiology of sarcoidosis.

There does appear to be geographic and racial clustering of sarcoidosis. The disease is very common in Scandinavia (60 people in every 100,000) and in Irish women in England. The disease is rare in Japan and rarely reported in areas of the world where tuberculosis is common. In the United States, sarcoidosis is more prevalent in African-Americans than Caucasians and more frequently seen in women. The disease usually manifests itself in people ages 20 to 40.

57. How is sarcoidosis diagnosed?

Sarcoidosis is diagnosed by three sets of findings:
- Lung biopsy that shows the presence of noncaseating granulomas
- Physical examination
- Ruling out of other granulomatous diseases

Granulomas can occur in almost any organ or tissue of the body. The lungs are one of the organs most commonly involved. Usually the granulomas will resolve spontaneously without damaging the underlying lung tissue, but in about 20% of patients pulmonary fibrosis develops.

58. What are the common signs and symptoms associated with sarcoidosis?

The common clinical symptoms are divided into three categories: dermatology, ophthalmology, and pulmonary. Lupus pernio and erythema nodosum are skin lesions associated with the disease. Common eye problems include conjunctival lesions, uveitis, excessive tearing, and, in chronic sarcoidosis, glaucoma and cataracts. Persistent dry cough, hemoptysis, hoarseness, dyspnea, wheezing, nasal congestion, and chest pain are the common pulmonary symptoms.

59. Describe the radiographic findings in sarcoidosis.

An abnormal chest x-ray can be found in 90% of the patients with sarcoidosis. Typically, bilateral hilar adenopathy and infiltrates are seen. In severe stages of the disease, fibrotic changes with honeycombing are present.

60. Describe the radiographic staging of sarcoidosis.

The radiographic staging includes:
- Stage 0: normal
- Stage 1: bilateral hilar adenopathy
- Stage 2: bilateral hilar adenopathy with infiltrates
- Stage 3: infiltrates

While helpful in the management of the disease, the staging process is also predictive of the course of the illness. Up to 80% of patients at the time of diagnosis with stage 1 disease have spontaneous resolution of the disease. Stage 2 patients see a spontaneous recovery of up to 60% and stage 3 only 20%.

61. What pulmonary function test abnormalities are seen in patients with sarcoidosis?

Pulmonary function tests (PFTs) are not used to definitively diagnose lung involvement in sarcoidosis. Frequently patients with mild sarcoidosis have normal PFT findings. In patients with more severe disease, a restrictive pattern is seen. The patient will have diminished lung volumes, a decrease in lung compliance, and diffusing capacity. In mild cases the patient will have hypoxia with exertion and eventually at rest as the disease becomes more severe. Serial spirometry is helpful in following the course of the patient's disease and in evaluating the effectiveness of medical therapy.

62. What is the treatment for sarcoidosis?

The primary intervention used in the treatment of sarcoidosis is steroid therapy. Stage 1 patients generally do not require treatment. Patients in stages 2 and 3 are generally treated unless they are asymptomatic and have stable/mildly impaired PFTs. Stage 2 and 3 patients must be monitored closely to ensure that their condition does not deteriorate in spite of medical therapy. These patients are usually started on prednisone taper therapy beginning at 30 to 60 mg/day. Serial PFTs are monitored closely, and the patient is reassessed at regular intervals for return of their original symptoms. Relapse is common during the steroid taper. Some patients may not be able to completely taper off of prednisone therapy. Other medications that can be used include methotrexate, azathioprine, and chloroquine. Topical steroids can be used to treat skin lesions and uveitis. Organ transplants, including lung, heart, kidney, and liver, have been used in a few patients with severe disease.

63. What is the prognosis associated with sarcoidosis?

Most patients will be symptom-free with no chest x-ray abnormalities within 2 years. Approximately 20% of the patients develop irreversible pulmonary fibrosis or airway narrowing. The mortality from sarcoidosis is less than 8%, and death usually occurs from pulmonary insufficiency and cor pulmonale.

64. What is pulmonary hypertension?

Pulmonary hypertension exists when the pressure in the pulmonary vascular bed is consistently elevated above a mean pressure of 30 mm Hg.

65. What are some of the risk factors associated with pulmonary hypertension?

Pulmonary hypertension usually occurs secondary to another preexisting illness. Patients at risk for developing secondary pulmonary hypertension are those with intracardiac shunting, cardiomyopathy, emphysema, scleroderma, lupus erythematosus, pulmonary embolism, sickle cell disease, or sleep apnea. When an underlying cause for the pulmonary hypertension cannot be identified, it is referred to as idiopathic or primary pulmonary hypertension (PPH).

66. What are the early signs and symptoms associated with pulmonary hypertension?

Typically, a patient with pulmonary hypertension has very few symptoms until the disease is well advanced. The pulmonary vasculature is able to accommodate large increases in pulmonary blood flow before the patient or health care provider notices symptoms. Fatigue and dyspnea on exertion are usually the complaints that bring a patient to seek medical attention. These general symptoms can frequently be attributed to being anxious, overworked, or physically unfit. Untreated, there is 45% to 50% mortality at 2 to 3 years after the onset of symptoms.

67. What are the later signs and symptoms associated with pulmonary hypertension?

As the disease progresses, the patient may complain of chest pain, syncope or presyncope, hemoptysis, hoarseness, and symptoms of right heart failure such as peripheral edema, the development of third or fourth heart sounds, and arterial hypoxemia that does not respond well to oxygen supplementation.

68. **What is the definitive diagnostic test in the evaluation of pulmonary hypertension?**

The only definitive test for pulmonary hypertension is a right heart catheterization.

69. **What other diagnostic testing may be used?**

- Pulmonary function test
- Echocardiogram
- Chest x-ray
- CT scan

70. **Describe the treatment of pulmonary hypertension.**

Treatment of pulmonary hypertension includes the use of supplemental oxygen. This helps to control the patient's hypoxia and reduce afterload on the right ventricle. Anticoagulation is necessary to prevent the development of venous thrombus and pulmonary embolism. Vasodilator therapy is also used in the treatment of pulmonary hypertension. This therapy is not very effective in patients with secondary pulmonary hypertension. Oral medications such as nifedipine and diltiazem are typically used. In patients with primary pulmonary hypertension (PPH), Flolan (epoprostenol), a potent intravenous vasodilator, can be used. Lung transplantation can occasionally be used as a treatment for pulmonary hypertension when all other therapies have been exhausted.

71. **What is Flolan and what is its mechanism of action?**

Flolan is a prostacyclin that is used in the treatment of primary pulmonary hypertension (PPH). Flolan mimics the effects of naturally occurring prostacyclin but has a very short half-life of 3 to 5 minutes and therefore must be administered in a continuous intravenous form via a central line. Initiation of the medication is done in the cardiac catheterization lab/intensive care unit, and titration of the dose is performed slowly over several weeks to months.

72. **What are the common side effects and problems associated with the use of Flolan?**

Most complaints from patients on Flolan occur with the initiation of therapy and with dose increases. Jaw pain, facial flushing, diarrhea, and headaches are the most common complaints. These symptoms generally resolve within a few days of dose adjustment. Line infection and breakage are long-term problems frequently seen with Flolan patients. Frequent or prolonged manipulation of the catheter and site can result in line sepsis or breakage and the need for catheter replacement. The drug is very unstable and once mixed with diluent must be kept refrigerated. While being infused the drug must be stored on ice packs.

73. Describe the cost issues associated with Flolan use.

The yearly cost of Flolan is between $50,000 and $100,000 depending on the patient's dosage.

74. What are the desired results of Flolan therapy?

Ideally, a decrease in the patient's pulmonary pressures should be seen with an increase in the Flolan dose. Frequently, the reduction in these pressures is not as significant as might be expected, although the patient's 6-minute walk test, pulmonary vascular resistance, and cardiac output are improved. It has been suggested that chronic use of Flolan also has nonvasodilating effects such as inotropy and vascular remodeling.

75. What other pharmacological alternatives are available to the patient with pulmonary hypertension?

Tracleer (bosentan) is a recently approved oral agent for the treatment of pulmonary hypertension. Tracleer blocks the action of endothelin, a naturally occurring substance in the body that causes narrowing of blood vessels and thus elevation in pulmonary pressures. Tracleer can be used in patients with mild PPH and in patients with secondary pulmonary hypertension. The two major risks when using this medication are the risk of liver toxicity and the drug's potential damage to a fetus. The drug is started at a half-dosage of 62.5 mg twice a day and increased to 125 mg twice a day after the first month if liver enzyme elevation is not present. The primary tools used to assess the effectiveness of Tracleer are the 6-minute walk test, CT scan, monitoring of liver enzymes, and the patient's subjective reporting. Tracleer is only slightly less expensive than Flolan but does not have the risks of a continuous infusion associated with it.

Remodulin is a synthetic form of prostacyclin that can be delivered subcutaneously. It is a more stable form of prostacyclin than Flolan with a half-life of 4 to 6 hours. It is delivered via an infusion pump through a subcutaneous needle, usually inserted in the abdomen. The side effects of Remodulin are similar to those of Flolan: headache, diarrhea, jaw pain, and flushing, but the patient may also complain of pain at the needle insertion site. The risk of line infection and sepsis seen with Flolan is less with Remodulin.

Beraprost and **Iloprost** are oral and inhaled forms, respectively, of prostacyclin currently being investigated.

76. What is a primary pneumothorax?

A primary pneumothorax is also referred to as a simple pneumothorax. A primary pneumothorax occurs abruptly as a result of rupture of a bleb or cyst in the apical lung region.

77. How does a pneumothorax develop?

A pneumothorax occurs when air enters the normally gas-free pleural space. The pleural space is located between the visceral pleura and the parietal pleura.

Normally this space contains a small amount of pleural fluid (5 to 15 ml). The pleural fluid serves as a lubricant between the two pleura. Pleural pressure is normally slightly negative as compared to atmospheric pressure. When the pleural space is penetrated, it is exposed to positive atmospheric pressure. This causes the lung to collapse inward. The underlying cause of the pneumothorax determines the severity of the pneumothorax and its symptoms and treatment.

78. Describe the typical patient that develops a primary pneumothorax.

The typical patient is a young male age 20 to 35. The patient is usually tall and slender in build and in good health. About 30% of these patients will have a reoccurrence within 3 years.

79. What are the common signs and symptoms associated with a primary pneumothorax?

The signs and symptoms of a primary pneumothorax are directly related to the size of the pneumothorax. A small pneumothorax that raises the intrapleural pressure only slightly will cause little in the way of symptoms and will be well tolerated by an otherwise healthy patient. With a larger pneumothorax, the patient will typically complain of sudden-onset pain that is pleuritic in nature. This pain lessens as air accumulates in the pleural space and separation of the pleural linings is complete. Eventually the character of the pain becomes a chronic dull ache. The patient will be tachycardic and short of breath. Auscultation of breath sounds will reveal diminished or absent breath sounds on the affected side.

80. What are some of the ECG findings associated with a pneumothorax?

An ECG may show signs that can be misinterpreted as a subendocardial myocardial infarction: decreased voltage, axis shifts, and T wave inversion across the pericardium.

81. How is the diagnosis of primary pneumothorax made?

The diagnosis of a primary pneumothorax is made from the patient's medical history, physical examination, and radiographic studies. The chest x-ray will show a partially collapsed lung outlined by the visceral pleural line. An end-expiratory chest film or a decubitus film may be needed to help visualize a small pneumothorax.

82. How is a pneumothorax treated?

If the pneumothorax is small (less than 20%) and the patient is asymptomatic, the patient does not require any treatment other than observation. The pneumothorax will reabsorb within 1 to 2 weeks. Intervention is required for a pneumothorax greater than 20%. A chest tube is inserted and connected to water seal/suction. A chest x-ray should be obtained to confirm correct placement of the chest tube. The chest tube is left in place until evidence of an air leak has been absent for at least 24 hours and the lung appears reexpanded on chest x-ray. In patients where this therapy is not effective or who have reoccurrence of the pneumothorax, additional surgical interventions may be required.

83. Describe other options in the treatment of a pneumothorax.

The goal of an invasive/surgical intervention is to irritate the pleural tissue and cause the development of adhesions and scar tissue, thus preventing a future reoccurrence of a pneumothorax. One option is to introduce a sclerosing agent (tetracycline) into the pleural space via the chest tube. This is a very painful procedure. Another alternative is thoracoscopic examination of the lung and pleura. General anesthesia is required for this procedure, but it allows direct examination of the chest to detect air leaks and blebs and to initiate repair. Pleurodesis can also be done via a thoracoscopic procedure. Pleurodesis is the mechanical irritation of the pleura so that scar tissue develops and prevents a future pneumothorax. Chemicals, talc, or pleural abrasion are examples of ways to mechanically stimulate the development of scar tissue.

84. What is a secondary or complicated spontaneous pneumothorax?

A secondary pneumothorax occurs in patients with underlying pulmonary disease. Some diseases in which a pneumothorax can be seen include COPD, interstitial fibrosis, neoplasm, infection, and *Pneumocystis carinii* pneumonia.

85. Describe the difference in managing a primary versus a secondary pneumothorax.

The diagnosis is made using the same set of criteria as previously described, and treatment is similar. The major difference between the two types of pneumothorax is that a patient with a secondary pneumothorax, because of their underlying disease, must be identified and treated quickly. These patients tend to have less pulmonary and cardiac reserve and can rapidly deteriorate to a life-threatening situation. In patients who are being mechanically ventilated, adjustment of the ventilator to high frequency, low pressure may be necessary to manage the air leak(s) and prevent further exacerbation.

86. Describe some additional causes of pneumothorax.

Trauma to the chest is another cause of a pneumothorax, either penetrating or nonpenetrating trauma. Typical sources for this type of pneumothorax are rib fractures, stab/bullet wounds, or deceleration injury to the chest such as occurs from an automobile accident.

An **iatrogenic pneumothorax** is seen as a complication associated with subclavian line placement, thoracentesis, or transbronchial lung biopsy.

A **catamenial pneumothorax** can occur in women with endometriosis. It typically occurs in women under the age of 30 and on the right side of the chest. A spontaneous pneumothorax occurs within 48 hours of the start of menstruation and is attributed to minute endometrial implants on the surface of the lung. Treatment includes ovulation-suppressing drugs and chemical pleurodesis.

87. What physiological changes occur in a patient with tension pneumothorax?

In a tension pneumothorax, air is allowed to continuously enter the pleural space. This causes an accumulation of positive pressure within the pleural space and significant lung collapse. If extreme, there can be shifting of the trachea and mediastinum to the contralateral side and even collapse of the uninvolved lung. The patient will exhibit hypotension and hemodynamic instability. This situation is a medical emergency and requires immediate intervention with a chest tube. If the patient is being mechanically ventilated at the time of the tension pneumothorax, the situation is even more urgent. Mechanical ventilation will only serve to increase the positive pressure within the pleural space and exacerbate the patient's symptoms.

88. What is idiopathic pulmonary fibrosis?

Idiopathic pulmonary fibrosis (IPF) is a chronic inflammatory process of the lung resulting in permanent destruction of lung tissue. IPF can occur as an isolated pulmonary process or in association with a collagen vascular disease such as rheumatoid arthritis or scleroderma. IPF is a rare disease occurring in people between the ages of 50 and 70 and affecting men more frequently than women. The life expectancy of someone diagnosed with IPF is about 5 years. Death is usually caused by respiratory failure and/or cor pulmonale.

89. What is the cause of IPF?

There are many known factors that contribute to IPF but no specific known cause. Environmental factors such as exposure to asbestos, metal dust, or organic materials found on farms (hay or mold), referred to as Farmer's lung, have been implicated in the development of IPF. Sarcoidosis, radiation therapy to the chest, collagen diseases, and genetic/familial history are also factors associated with pulmonary fibrosis. The term IPF is used when all known causes of the pulmonary fibrosis have been ruled out.

90. What is the diagnostic work-up for a person with suspected IPF?

Patient history: Dyspnea is the patient complaint that most commonly causes the patient to seek medical advice. The patient may also complain of a chronic dry cough.

Physical exam: On physical examination the patient will have rapid, shallow breathing; end-inspiratory crackles in the lung bases; and in later stages of the disease, clubbing of the fingers and symptoms of pulmonary hypertension.

Arterial blood gas analysis: Arterial blood gas analysis initially shows hypoxemia during exercise, and as the disease progresses, hypoxemia will occur while the patient is at rest. Because of the lung's increasing noncompliance, hyperventilation is its response to hypoxemia and exertion.

Pulmonary function tests (PFTs): PFTs show a decrease in lung compliance and lung volume.

Chest x-ray: In the early stages of IPF, the chest x-ray appears normal. Later on, bilateral infiltrates most pronounced in the bases are seen.

CT scan of the chest: A CT scan of the chest will reveal honeycombing. A CT scan is more helpful than a chest x-ray in identifying IPF and its progression.

Lung biopsy: An open lung biopsy is needed for a definitive diagnosis of IPF. Tissue samples from at least two sites are preferable. Biopsy done by bronchoscopy or a bronchoalveolar lavage is not as useful because of the patchy nature of the lung disease and the inability to obtain an adequate tissue sample. The histology results from a biopsy can be placed into one of several categories. The most common are UIP (usual interstitial pneumonitis) and DIP (desquamative interstitial pneumonitis).

91. What is the treatment for IPF?

Currently, there is no cure for IPF. Medical treatment is focused on the use of steroids to minimize the inflammatory process of the disease. Prednisone at 1.5 mg/kg per day in combination with an immunosuppressive agent such as azathioprine is one treatment regimen. It may be as long as 6 to 9 months before positive results can be seen. Serial PFTs and CT scans should be done to monitor the progress of the disease. Quite frequently lifelong maintenance therapy is required. Interferon gamma-1b is also being used in the treatment of IPF for patients who do not respond to steroid and immunosuppressive therapy. This medication is given in conjunction with steroids as a subcutaneous injection 3 times a week. The patients must be taught how to self-administer the injection. A family member must also be taught the procedure. The primary side effect from the medication is flulike symptoms. These symptoms can be very debilitating but should become minimal over time. To cope with these side effects, the patient is instructed to premedicate with Tylenol and administer the medication before bedtime.

Other options include:
- Pulmonary rehabilitation
- Oxygen therapy
- Pneumococcal vaccine
- Influenza vaccine
- Transplantation

Key Points

- COPD is a disease characterized by airflow limitations. The disease states include emphysema and chronic bronchitis.
- An estimated 50,000 patients will die from pneumonia annually.
- Common symptoms associated with tuberculosis include anorexia, night sweats, fever, weight loss, and hemoptysis.

Internet Resources

American Thoracic Society: Assembly History:
http://www.thoracic.org/assemblies/nur/nur4a.asp

Medfacts: Management of Chronic Obstructive Pulmonary Disease (COPD):
http://www.njc.org/medfacts/management.html

CHEST:
http://www.chestjournal.org

BIBLIOGRAPHY

American Thoracic Society: Statement on sarcoidosis, *Am J Respir Crit Care Med* 160:739-755, 1999.

American Thoracic Society: International consensus statement on idiopathic pulmonary fibrosis: diagnosis and treatment, *Am J Respir Crit Care Med* 161:646-664, 2000.

Bordow RA, Ries AL, Morris TA, editors: *Manual of Clinical Problems in Pulmonary Medicine*, ed 5, Philadelphia, 2001, Lippincott, Williams & Wilkins.

Fishman AP, editor: *Pulmonary Diseases and Disorders Companion Handbook*, ed 2, New York, 1994, McGraw-Hill.

Hanson D, Winterbauer RII, Kirtland SII, Wu R: Changes in pulmonary function test results after one year of therapy as predictors of survival in patients with idiopathic pulmonary fibrosis, *Chest* 108:305-310, Aug 1995.

Hayes DD: Stemming the tide of pleural effusion, *Nursing* 31(5):49-52, 2001.

Hayes GB: *Pulmonary Hypertension—A Patient's Survival Guide*, 2004, Pulmonary Hypertension Association, Silver Spring, Maryland.

Rubin LJ, Badesch DB, Barst RJ, Galie N, Black CM, Keogh A, Pulido T, Frost A, Roux S, Leconte I, Landzberg M, Simonneau G: Bosentan therapy for pulmonary arterial hypertension, *N Engl J Med* 346:896-903, March 2002.

Ziesche R, Hofbauer E, Wittman K, Petkov V, Block LH: A preliminary study of long-term treatment with interferon gamma-1b and low-dose prednisolone in patients with idiopathic pulmonary fibrosis, *N Engl J Med* 341:1264-1269, Oct 1999.

Thoracic Surgical Procedures

Janice Jones

1. **What is the primary function of the thorax?**

   The thorax is the portion of the body below the neck and above the diaphragm. The change in volume of the thoracic cavity during inspiration and expiration is the primary factor influencing the mechanics of breathing. During inspiration the thorax is actively enlarged by coordinated muscle contractions. Contraction of the diaphragm and intercostal muscles expands the thoracic cavity, resulting in a reduction in intrathoracic, intrapleural, and intrapulmonic pressures that forces atmospheric air into the lungs. During expiration relaxation of the force produced during inspiration allows air to passively exit the lungs. This is marked by the return of the thoracic pressures to resting levels.

2. **What is the structural support of the thorax?**

   The thorax includes the sternum, 10 pairs of ribs and costal cartilage, 2 pairs of ribs without cartilage, and 12 thoracic vertebra and intervertebral disks. The intercostal space consists of three layers of muscle and deep fascia. From superficial to deep, the muscle layers are: external intercostals; internal intercostals and fascia; innermost intercostals, subcostals, and transverse thoracic muscles. The inferior structural support for the thorax is the diaphragm, which is separated into the the right and left hemidiaphragm.

3. **What purpose does the diaphragm have?**

   The diaphragm is the major muscle of inspiration. Its alternating contraction and relaxation cause pressure changes in the thoracic cavity that aid in inspiration and expiration. The diaphragm also serves as the anatomic division between the thoracic and abdominopelvic cavities. While the diaphragm is innervated by the phrenic nerves, the internal and external intercostal muscles are innervated by the intercostal nerves. Damage to any of these nerves can result in paralysis of the diaphragm.

4. **How are the lobes of the lungs divided?**

The right lung has three lobes (upper, middle, and lower) and two fissures (major and minor). The left lung has two lobes (upper and lower) and one fissure. The left lung is smaller than the right so that it can accommodate the heart, which is situated slightly to the left of the median plane. The cardiac notch is a concavity in the left lung that surrounds the heart. Also found on the left lung is the lingula (lingula pulmonis sinistri); this tonguelike projection is located in a position comparable to the right middle lobe and serves as an anatomical landmark.

5. **In which lung field is aspiration pneumonia most likely to occur?**

Aspiration pneumonia typically occurs in the right lung because of the anatomical structure of the bronchial tree. The trachea bifurcates at the level of T7 into the right and left mainstem bronchi. Because the right mainstem bronchus is shorter, wider, and more directly in line with the trachea, it is a more common site for aspiration pneumonia. A major anatomical landmark of the trachea is the carina; this piece of cartilage projects posteriorly from the trachea at the point where it bifurcates into the mainstem bronchi.

6. **What are the three compartments of the mediastinum?**

The mediastinum can be divided into three compartments: anterior, middle, and posterior. The anterior mediastinum can be subdivided into anterior and superior portions. The anterior mediastinum is located in the anterior pericardium. The middle mediastinum is situated between the anterior portion of the pericardium and the anterior portion of the vertebral body. The posterior mediastinum lies in between the anterior and posterior portions of the vertebral body.

7. **Outline the lymphatic system of the lungs.**

The lymphatic system of the lungs includes the intrapulmonary and the mediastinal lymph nodes. The intrapulmonary lymph nodes are found beneath visceral pleura in connective tissue. The mediastinal nodes are within the mediastinum and are classified as nodal stations 1-10.

8. **What are the different categories of mediastinal lymph nodes?**

The mediastinal lymph nodes are separated into four categories: the paratracheal nodes, the tracheobronchial nodes, the posterior mediastinal nodes, and the anterior mediastinal nodes. Within the tracheobronchial nodes is station 7, which is the subcarinal location, an important nodal station. The nodal stations are important when staging lung cancers.

9. **During the preoperative surgical examination, what information should be obtained from a patient scheduled for thoracic surgery?**

In addition to a general medical and surgical history, the examination should focus more specifically on pulmonary history. Some important information that

should be obtained is:
- History of asthma
- History of chronic obstructive pulmonary disease (COPD)
- History of pneumonia
- Smoking history
- TB exposure/history
- Cough, with or without sputum production
- Fever, chills
- Shortness of breath
- Dyspnea on exertion
- Pain
- Weight loss/gain
- Exposure to environmental toxins or chemicals
- Travel out of the country
- Family history of pulmonary diseases such as cystic fibrosis

10. **What is the importance of a computed tomography (CT) scan of the thorax?**

A CT scan helps determine the size and location of the lung pathology. A CT scan with contrast will provide more details regarding the mediastinum and soft tissues in the thorax. This diagnostic test can be used to evaluate interstitial lung disease, emphysema, parenchyma, and mediastinal tumors or abnormalities.

11. **When assessing the resectability of a pulmonary lesion, which tests should be ordered?**

To determine whether a patient is a candidate for pulmonary resection and to assess general pulmonary risk after surgery, a pulmonary function test (PFT) and a quantitative ventilation/perfusion (VQ) scan should be ordered. The PFT will measure airflow, lung volume, lung mechanics, and gas exchange. The VQ scan will assess ventilation and perfusion to all areas of the lungs, including the different regions.

12. **When evaluating a patient scheduled for pulmonary resection, which PFT value is most important?**

The forced expiratory volume in 1 second (FEV_1) is assessed most frequently by surgeons when evaluating a patient for pulmonary nodule resection. The FEV_1 is a percent of the forced vital capacity (FVC). To determine if a patient will tolerate a portion of lung removed, the FEV_1 should not fall below 0.8 L after the resection. With the addition of the VQ scan this can be determined. An estimated postoperative FEV_1 less than 0.8 L may preclude a patient from consideration for surgical resection.

13. **How is measurement of arterial blood gas used to determine pulmonary risk for surgery?**

An arterial blood gas (ABG) measurement can be used to help determine a patient's pulmonary risk for any surgical intervention. Hypercarbia or a $PaCO_2$ >45 mm Hg is a direct indicator of advanced lung disease. These patients will have minimal pulmonary reserve and may have a difficult postoperative course.

14. What are preoperative indications for a bronchoscopy?

Bronchoscopy, either flexible or rigid, can be used to help diagnose pulmonary lesions by bronchial washing or needle biopsy. Bronchoscopy can also determine if a lesion is within the bronchial tree. Another use for bronchoscopy is to clear secretions. In addition, bronchoscopy can be employed to evaluate the origin of hemoptysis and then control it.

15. What is the purpose of a positron emission tomography (PET) scan?

PET scans can help determine if a nodule found on a CT scan is highly suspicious for cancer. The scan will appear lighter in areas of increased uptake of FDG (Fludeoxyglucose), an isotope. If the PET scan correlates with the CT scan, then the nodule is suspicious for cancer. However, it must be noted that the PET scan will also appear lighter in areas of infection or active metabolism.

16. What are indications for mediastinoscopy?

Mediastinoscopy is indicated for use in the clinical staging of lung cancer, which most commonly spreads via the paratracheal lymph nodes. Mediastinoscopy can also be used to diagnose mediastinal and hilar adenopathy of unknown etiology, such as sarcoidosis and lymphoma. Mediastinoscopy has a sensitivity of approximately 74% and a specificity of approximately 94%.

17. What testing is needed before mediastinoscopy?

The most important diagnostic test before mediastinoscopy is a CT scan with or without contrast. This will show the location and size of the mass or adenopathy and will also evaluate the surrounding structures. Depending on the diagnosis and the patient's history, PFTs may need to be performed. On CT scan, if the mass causes a decrease in tracheal cross section >35%, surgery is contraindicated or is considered high-risk because of the potential for the mass to cause tracheal obstruction upon induction of anesthesia.

18. How is mediastinoscopy performed?

Mediastinoscopy is performed under general anesthesia, with the patient intubated. A small incision is made 2 cm above the sternal notch along the anterior surface of the trachea (4-cm transverse incision). A lighted hollow tube is then passed behind the sternum, allowing biopsy of the mediastinal lymph nodes. This is usually a same-day procedure.

19. What areas of the mediastinum are contraindicated for mediastinoscopy?

Mediastinoscopy cannot reach the anterior mediastinum, the aortopulmonary window, or the posterior subcarinal area. An anterior thoracotomy access is needed for evaluation of the anterior mediastinum and the aortopulmonary window area.

20. What are some potential complications of mediastinoscopy?

The mortality of mediastinoscopy is approximately 0.1%; however, it does have some potential complications. Hemorrhage is a possibility because of the close proximity of great vessels. If this should occur, median sternotomy should be performed to gain hemostatic control. Infection can also occur after mediastinoscopy. Pneumothorax and injury to the recurrent laryngeal nerve are also potential complications.

21. What are contraindications to mediastinoscopy?

In some patients with large anteriosuperior and middle mediastinal masses, mediastinoscopy is contraindicated because of the potential for cardiovascular and respiratory compromise. The loss of negative intrathoracic pressure, the relaxation of bronchial smooth muscles, or a decrease in tidal volume from placing these patients under general anesthesia may result in extrinsic airway compression.

22. What are indications for thoracentesis?

Thoracentesis can be performed for numerous reasons. One reason is to diagnose a pleural effusion of unknown etiology. Thoracentesis can also be used for the relief of symptoms associated with a pleural effusion. Therefore it can be performed for diagnostic or therapeutic purposes.

23. Before performing a thoracentesis, what diagnostic studies should be executed?

Before a thoracentesis, either an ultrasound or a CT scan can be used to locate the effusion. Guidance by CT or ultrasound can be particularly helpful if the effusion is loculated (fluid surrounded by a capsule). Thoracentesis can also be done at bedside. Percussion is used to determine the placement of the needle. The needle is then placed approximately 2 inches below the area of dullness.

24. What is the definition of an exudative pleural effusion?

To determine if a pleural fluid is exudative, fluid obtained via thoracentesis should be sent to a microbiology lab for evaluation. The fluid is studied for protein and L-lactate dehydrogenase (LDH). For fluid to be exudative one of the following criteria must be met:
  • Pleural fluid protein to serum protein ratio >0.5
  • Pleural fluid LDH to serum LDH ratio >0.6
  • Pleural fluid LDH $>\frac{2}{3}$ upper limit of serum LDH
Exudates tend to be infectious in origin. Transudative effusions meet none of the above criteria.

25. What are indications for pleurodesis?

Pleurodesis is used in the treatment of pneumothorax and chronic or malignant pleural effusions. For pneumothorax treatment it is indicated when an air leak is persistent for over 7 days, if it is the second occurrence of a pneumothorax, or if it is the first occurrence in a patient with one lung. In patients with a pleural effusion, it is indicated when patients have rapid reaccumulation of fluid after thoracentesis.

26. What are the different ways pleurodesis can be performed?

Pleurodesis can be done bedside with sclerosing agents such as silver nitrate, talc, doxycycline, or hypertonic glucose. It can also be done in the operating room under general anesthesia with single lung ventilation. This method, mostly used for pneumothorax, uses either mechanical abrasion or bleb resection, or both. With either therapy, a chest tube is needed.

27. What are indications for video-assisted thoracoscopy (VATS) and thoracotomy?

VATS and thoracotomy can be used for diagnostic or therapeutic purposes. Examples of diagnostic purposes are for the diagnosis of pleural effusion exudate and for tissue diagnosis of either pleural-based or lung-based mediastinal lymph nodes or mediastinal masses. Therapeutic uses of VATS and thoracotomy are for pleurodesis, bullectomy, lung cancer resection, esophageal surgery, mediastinal resection, bronchogenic cyst resection, or empyema.

28. What is the difference between VATS and thoracotomy?

VATS uses minimal incisions with the aid of a videoscope to perform thoracic surgery. Two or three small incisions are made, one for the video camera and one for the long instruments needed to perform the surgery. Thoracotomy requires a longer incision and allows direct visualization of the surgical area. Both techniques are performed through the rib spaces.

29. What are limitations associated with VATS?

Limitations to using a VATS procedure are associated with access and visualization of the surgical area as well as compliance with the lungs. When attempting to biopsy very small pulmonary lesions, deep parenchymal lesions, or hilar lesions, a thoracotomy is recommended to provide better access. In patients with severe emphysema, in ventilator-dependent patients, or for patients with non-compliant lung tissue, thoracotomy is again recommended to provide better access and control during surgery.

30. What are potential complications/disadvantages associated with VATS?

VATS uses long instruments with the aid of a video camera to access the surgical site. There is a learning curve associated with performing surgery this way.

Incomplete staging of lung cancer can occur as a result of the limited access with VATS. If there is excessive bleeding during a VATS, it will be very difficult to control and the procedure may need to be modified to a thoracotomy. A pneumothorax may occur after the procedure. Potential infection is always a concern.

31. What are the different types of thoracotomy incisions?

There are multiple types of thoracotomy incisions: anterior, posterolateral, axillary, and median sternotomy. The type of incision used depends on the procedure being performed and the location of the surgical area. Regardless of the incision, either one or two chest tubes are placed postoperatively to remove excess fluid and air. The same is true for VATS.

32. What are the potential complications associated with a thoracotomy?

Thoracotomy and VATS have similar complications. Damage to a major blood vessel can result; however, bleeding will be easier to control with the larger incision of a thoracotomy. Pneumothorax or infection can also occur. Depending on the procedure, cardiac arrhythmias or spinal cord injury may also develop.

33. What is meant by an open lung biopsy?

An open lung biopsy is a direct surgical approach that provides access to large amounts of lung tissue. This technique is done under general anesthesia, with a thoracotomy approach. Portions of both the involved and the uninvolved lung are sampled. Open biopsy is used in the diagnosis of diffuse infiltrates; the specimen usually undergoes histology, microbiology, and other microscopic studies.

34. What is bullous lung disease?

A bleb is a well-circumscribed intrapleural air space separated from the underlying parenchyma by a thin pleural covering. Bullous lung disease is more common in the upper lobes; however, it can be present in any area of the lungs.

35. What are indications for surgical removal of a bulla?

There are a few reasons why a bullectomy should be performed. Patients with bullous lung disease are more likely to suffer a pneumothorax. In these patients bullectomy is performed to decrease the incidence of a recurrent pneumothorax. Bullae can also become infected. If it fails to respond to medical therapy, surgical removal is warranted. Other indications are hemoptysis, suspicion of lung cancer, or chest pain, which may be related to air trapped in the area of the bullae.

36. What preoperative tests and treatments should be done before a bullectomy?

Before undergoing a bullectomy a CT scan should be performed. This not only will provide the location and size of the bulla but also will show the degree of underlying emphysema, which is usually present. Pulmonary function tests are usually not needed because most true bullae do not contribute to ventilation. However, if diffuse emphysema is present, PFTs and a VQ scan should be performed to assess the degree of emphysema. No single test is an absolute predictor of postoperative recovery/success. Before a bullectomy the patient should be optimized medically to reverse airway obstruction and bronchospasm and to control infection.

37. **What are surgical considerations in a bullectomy?**

A bullectomy is the surgical removal of a bulla. This procedure is done under general anesthesia. The patient is required to have single lung ventilation; therefore a double lumen endotracheal tube is used. The lung on the operative side is deflated; the bullous portion of the lung is removed using a stapling device. Most bullectomies are done via a posterolateral thoracotomy or VATS approach. A chest tube is placed to allow evacuation of air and fluid postoperatively. If bullous lung disease is bilateral, staging of operations is done.

38. **What are potential postoperative complications of a bullectomy?**

Because a bulla by definition is a weakened area of lung tissue, air leaks may be common postoperatively. Emphysematous lung tissue takes longer to heal than healthy tissue. If the patient is on steroids preoperatively, they should be discontinued if possible. A pneumothorax can develop postoperatively if chest tubes are inadequate to remove excess air in the thoracic cavity. This could lead to a tension pneumothorax if not dealt with properly. Bleeding and infection at the incision site or lung can also occur postoperatively.

39. **What are indications for a pneumonectomy?**

Most patients have a pneumonectomy because of lung cancer. Other indications are bronchiectasis and occasionally tuberculosis.

40. **How are patients evaluated for a pneumonectomy?**

Patients are evaluated in the same way any thoracotomy patient is evaluated. A CT scan is needed to assess the location of the mass and the proximity to hilar structures. Pulmonary function tests and quantitative VQ scans are also needed to determine if a patient can tolerate using only one lung for ventilation and perfusion. The risk of death and the risk of reduction in exercise capacity are also important considerations before a pneumonectomy.

41. **What are some surgical concerns during a pneumonectomy?**

During a pneumonectomy a double-lumen endotracheal tube is used to allow collapse of the affected lung. Once the lung is separated from the bronchus, the stump is sutured to close the airway. When performing a left pneumonectomy, care must be taken not to injure the phrenic nerves. Mediastinal shifting is another concern. In the postoperative period some surgeons aspirate air from the pleural space to bring the mediastinum to center, or they may place a chest tube to "balance" the mediastinum.

42. **What should be considered in the management of the pleural space in a postpneumonectomy patient?**

Once the lung is removed from the affected side, an empty space is left. Some surgeons do not place a chest tube postoperatively in order to allow fluid to accumulate. A chest tube may be placed, however, to prevent mediastinal shifting. Following the procedure there will usually be elevation of the ipsilateral diaphragm, shifting of the mediastinum toward the opposite side, and narrowing of the intercostal spaces on the operative side.

Key Points

- The diaphragm is the major muscle of respiration.
- Coughing, deep breathing, and incentive spirometry are very important treatment modalities that help prevent postoperative complications.
- The most common reason for a pneumonectomy is lung cancer.

Internet Resources

Video Assisted Thoracic Surgery (VATS):
http://www.thoracicgroup.com/HTML/vatsmain.html

American Association for Thoracic Surgery:
http://www.aats.org

BIBLIOGRAPHY

Baumgartner FJ: *Cardiothoracic Surgery*, 1997, RG Landes and Chapman & Hall, New York.

Criner GJ, D'Alonzo G: *Pulmonary Pathophysiology*, Madison, Connecticut, 1999, Fence Creek.

Ewald GA, McKenzie CR, editors: *Manual of Medical Therapeutics*, ed 28, Boston, 1995, Little, Brown and Co.

Lung Transplantation

Nancy Blumenthal

1. What are the indications for lung transplantation?

Lung transplantation is considered for patients with end-stage lung disease that have exhausted all other medical options. Diseases amenable to lung transplantation fall into four major categories: obstructive lung disease, fibrotic lung disease, septic lung disease, and vascular lung disease. The most common diagnoses in each category are listed below.

- Obstructive lung disease: emphysema, chronic obstructive pulmonary disease (COPD), alpha$_1$-antitrypsin deficiency
- Fibrotic lung disease: idiopathic pulmonary fibrosis, sarcoidosis
- Septic lung disease: cystic fibrosis, bronchiectasis
- Vascular lung disease: primary pulmonary hypertension, Eisenmenger's syndrome

2. Is lung transplantation considered an experimental procedure?

No. Lung transplantation is a proven therapy that has been available since the early 1980s for the treatment of end-stage lung disease.

3. What are contraindications to lung transplantation?

Patients must be free of life-threatening extrapulmonary diseases. Significant irreversible cardiac, renal, hepatic, or neurological impairment all confer poor outcomes following lung transplantation. Similarly, recent history of malignancy or active viral illness is considered a contraindication to transplantation. For some patients consultation by a specialist is required to predict the prognosis and course of the disease in the setting of post-transplant immunosuppression. Patients who demonstrate a history of substance abuse (including tobacco), medical noncompliance, or severe psychiatric illness warrant particular assessment as to their ability to follow the complex post-transplant self-care regimen. Comorbid conditions such as uncontrolled diabetes mellitus, symptomatic osteoporosis, significant obesity or cachexia, and profound debilitation detract from an individual's viability following this procedure and are considered relative contraindications.

4. **What is included in the evaluation of a candidate for lung transplantation?**

The studies and consultations included in a lung transplant evaluation are used to define the exact nature of an individual's lung disease and the impact it has on his or her overall health. The recommendations that stem from the evaluation not only determine a patient's suitability for transplantation but also may suggest alternate or related treatment options. Attention from multiple disciplines is required to ensure a patient is in the best condition while awaiting, undergoing, and recovering from lung transplant surgery. Though the assessment is tailored to the individual's history, the studies and consultations standard to lung transplant evaluation may include:

- Pulmonary function testing
- Arterial blood gas measurement
- Six-minute walk test
- Exercise desaturation study or full exercise study
- Quantitative ventilation-perfusion scan
- Chest x-ray
- Chest CT scan
- 12-lead ECG
- Echocardiogram
- Left and right heart catheterization
- 24-hour creatinine clearance
- Purified protein derivative (PPD) levels
- DEXA scan
- Blood work: comprehensive metabolic panel, complete blood count, coagulation studies, fasting lipid profile, blood typing, tissue typing, viral studies (HIV, herpes simplex virus [HSV], hepatitis B, hepatitis C, Epstein-Barr virus [EBV], cytomegalovirus [CMV])
- Pulmonary rehabilitation consultation
- Nutrition consultation
- Social work consultation
- Psychiatry consultation
- Transplant financing consultation
- Dental and gynecological clearance

5. **What factors determine whether a patient is listed for a unilateral or a bilateral lung transplant?**

Several factors can influence the decision as to the best procedure for a given patient. Surgical history, recipient age, native lung disease, and center-specific protocols are all taken into consideration. If a patient suffers from septic lung disease, bilateral (double-lung) transplant is required to prevent native lung infection from spreading to the allograft in the setting of post-transplant immunosuppression. For perioperative hemodynamic security, many centers prefer to perform bilateral lung transplant on patients with pulmonary hypertension. Unilateral (single-lung) transplant is the most common procedure for patients with pulmonary fibrosis or COPD because it maximizes the use of donor lungs (one donor can provide organs for two recipients) while still offering the recipient adequate pulmonary function to achieve quality-of-life goals.

Because single-lung transplant is less invasive than bilateral transplant, patients who are older or debilitated tolerate it better. Prior thoracic surgery, ventilation-perfusion distribution, and radiographic findings are all used to determine whether a patient is listed for a unilateral or bilateral lung transplant.

6. **How should a patient prepare for lung transplant surgery?**

- Follow medical recommendations identified during transplant evaluation.
- Attend regularly scheduled follow-up appointments with transplant team.
- Exercise regularly in a pulmonary rehabilitation program.
- Maintain or achieve optimal nutrition (that is, weight loss or gain) as advised by the transplant dietician.
- Immediately communicate all changes in condition (for example, medication changes or hospitalization) with lung transplant team.
- Identify a method for the transplant coordinator to contact the patient when the patient is not at home (for example, mobile phone or pager). The patient must be accessible AT ALL TIMES to avoid missing the call or jeopardizing the case. Be sure that the transplant team has accurate contact numbers.
- Get legal affairs in order: prepare a will, discuss advanced directives with surrogate medical decision maker.
- Confirm adequate insurance coverage of expected health care bills including prescriptions.
- Consider attending support groups offered for lung transplant patients and loved ones.
- Learn as much as possible about what to realistically expect of transplant process.
- Make arrangements for transportation to the hospital when called for transplant. It is very important that the mode of travel meet time constraints established by the transplant center and that the plan be effective at any time of day or in any weather conditions.
- If needed, have a plan for local housing for loved ones during the hospitalization and for the period of time following hospital discharge.

7. **What factors should be considered when choosing a lung transplant center?**

- Number of lung transplants performed
- Center-specific outcomes for patient's diagnosis
- Average waiting time
- Distance to transplant center and need to relocate
- Insurance coverage for specific center
- Accessibility of information and care from transplant team
- Availability of psychosocial support for patient and loved ones
- Patient's comfort with style of clinicians and staff at specific center
- Patient's ability to meet self-care and follow-up expectations of individual center

8. **Is the Internet a reliable source for information about lung transplantation?**

A great deal of information can be gathered in a patient-friendly fashion from many sites on the Internet. However, care must be taken to determine whether the content is accurate, thorough, current, and applicable to an individual's unique circumstances. Both lay people and professionals are encouraged to use sites that are refereed by experts and to confirm information with a clinician who is familiar with both the Internet site and the patient's care.

9. Can a patient get listed for lung transplantation at more than one center?

The nation's waiting list is subdivided into 11 regions within which donor lungs are allocated locally. UNOS regulations allow patients to list at only one center per region because there is only one waiting list per region. Provided that a patient can meet the clinical and practical requirements of different centers, he or she can list at as many centers as desired. This practice is discouraged by some centers and in some cases is not allowed.

10. How are donor lungs allocated in the United States?

The Organ Procurement and Transplantation Network (OPTN) was established by the United States government in 1984 to ensure a fair, safe, and effective process of solid organ donation, procurement, allocation, and transplantation. Shortly thereafter, the United Network for Organ Sharing (UNOS) was commissioned to operate the centralized computer network that links all organ procurement programs with all transplant centers in the country. The country is subdivided into 11 geographical regions within which local Organ Procurement Organizations (OPOs) facilitate donor activity. When a lung transplant candidate is placed on the waiting list, basic demographic information is entered into the UNOS database. The patient's diagnosis, blood type, and size are entered along with specific information about the organ that is needed (for example, right lung, left lung, either lung, or both lungs). The database is blind to the patient's age, race, ethnicity, faith, or financial status.

When a donor lung becomes available, the local OPO enters the donor's medical characteristics into the UNOS database. A list of locally registered ABO-compatible potential recipients is generated. The recipient names are listed according to time spent on the waiting list; that is, the longer a patient has been on the list, the closer they will be to the top of the list. Unlike other solid organ transplants, there is no status whereby medical urgency gives one patient priority over another. The clinical staff of the OPO then offers the lung to the clinician on call for the recipient lung transplant program. In that conversation, details regarding the donor's medical history, cause of death, hospitalization, pulmonary status, and hemodynamic stability are discussed. It is incumbent upon the transplant program staff to determine the suitability of a specific donor lung for a given recipient. Size, age, donor medical history, and recipient condition all factor into the clinical decision of whether the match is acceptable. If the lung is not suitable for the patient at the top of the list, it is then considered for the second patient on the list. This process continues until the local list is exhausted. If there are no recipients within the same region as the donor OPO, the offer is then extended, using the same criteria, to patients listed at centers within a 500-mile radius.

11. How is a potential lung donor evaluated?

Individuals who have been declared brain-dead in a hospital setting are considered potential organ donors. Once this diagnosis is established, the local OPO is notified. A member of the clinical staff of the OPO, an organ procurement coordinator, will then approach the next of kin to discuss the option of organ donation. If consent is granted, the procurement coordinator collaborates with the donor's clinical staff in the further direction of the donor's care. Emphasis is placed on evaluating and maximizing multiple organ function so that as many organs as possible can be placed.

Absolute contraindications to lung donation include active malignancy, communicable viral illness, and significant history of pulmonary disease. Age over 55 years, smoking history greater than 15 pack years, and endotracheal intubation for greater than 72 hours are all relative concerns and may influence the choice of a compatible recipient. The information communicated by the procurement staff to the lung transplant team includes:

- Cause of brain death
- Medical history
- Events of hospitalization
- Chest x-ray (within 2 hours and radiographic trends)
- Sputum culture and sensitivity
- Arterial blood gas trends
- "Oxygen challenge" arterial blood gas (within 2 hours and trends) on settings:
  - 100% fractional inspired oxygen concentration (FiO_2), +5 positive end-expiratory pressure (PEEP), tidal volume of 10 to 15 ml/kg for 20 minutes
- Hemodynamic data

12. Is it possible to have a living lung donor?

Yes. In very rare circumstances, one lower lobe can be taken from each of two healthy living donors for bilateral transplantation into a smaller recipient who might otherwise not survive the wait for a cadaveric (brain-dead) donor. To date, this procedure has been performed more commonly in the pediatric population. Because of the surgical risk associated with lobectomy in the donors, this remains a controversial option and is not widely practiced. Interestingly, recipient outcomes are comparable to those found in the cadaveric lung recipient.

13. What is an acceptable ischemic time for a pulmonary allograft?

Ischemic time begins when blood flow to the lung is stopped (that is, cross-clamp time) in the donor and ends when blood flow is resumed (that is, reperfusion) in the recipient. Ideally this takes less than 4 to 6 hours.

14. What factors influence ischemic time?

- Distance and travel time between the donor hospital and the recipient hospital
- Technical difficulty of explanting native recipient lung(s)

- Intraoperative hemodynamic stability
- Choice of procedure (for example, a second lung implanted in a bilateral sequential lung transplant sustains a longer ischemic time)

15. How is the donor lung surgically connected to the recipient's anatomy?

There are three anastamotic sites for each lung transplanted:
- Recipient mainstem bronchus to donor bronchus, overlapping donor bronchus by two to three cartilaginous rings; this provides blood flow to the anastamosis, which is necessary to prevent tissue necrosis and dehiscence
- Recipient pulmonary artery to donor pulmonary artery
- Donor pulmonary veins to recipient left atrial cuff

16. What is the difference between a double-lung transplant and a bilateral sequential transplant?

The term "bilateral sequential" describes the most common technique used for bilateral lung transplantation. Specifically, two single-lung transplants (one immediately following the other) are performed in the same operation. This technique requires single-lung ventilation of the lung contralateral to the surgical site, but allows for the procedure to be done without cardiopulmonary bypass. In a double-lung ("en bloc") transplant, the patient is supported on cardiopulmonary bypass while the native lungs are both removed and the donor lungs are implanted. The airway anastamosis in a double-lung procedure is at the level of the trachea, but the vascular connections are the same as described previously.

17. What are the immediate postoperative priorities of care?

- Hemodynamic support
- Optimizing gas exchange
- Pain management
- Infection prevention/control
- Immunosuppression

18. How does pulmonary care for a lung transplant recipient differ from that of other postoperative patients in the ICU?

The two principles that distinguish the care of a patient with pulmonary allografts are fluid balance and immunosuppression. As a result of ischemic injury, the capillary membrane has very low permeability. This makes the lung very susceptible to interstitial edema. The fluid balance goal is to minimize vascular congestion (right atrial pressure 3 to 6 mm Hg) while still maintaining adequate kidney perfusion (as measured by systemic blood pressure, serum creatinine, and urine output). Immunosuppression, necessitated by rejection prophylaxis, renders the recipient at increased risk for infection and sepsis. Recipients previously colonized with bacterial or fungal organisms may develop invasive disease. Nosocomial infections may develop from either the donor or the recipient ICUs.

Latent viruses can be reactivated in the setting of immunosuppression. Extra care must be taken to prevent, expeditiously recognize, and treat any infection in this medically vulnerable population.

19. **What complications can occur in the early post-transplant period?**
    * Hyperacute rejection (intraoperative)
    * Hemorrhage (perioperative)
    * Primary graft failure
    * Infection
    * Airway anastamotic compromise (for example, dehiscence, stenosis, malacia, infection)
    * Acute rejection
    * Cardiac arrhythmias

20. **What is a typical medication regimen after lung transplantation?**

    Though protocols vary from center to center, standard maintenance immuno-suppressive therapy is based on a three-drug regimen:
    * Corticosteroids (for example, prednisone, Solu-Medrol, Medrol, or Decadron)
    * Calcineurin inhibitors (for example, cyclosporine or tacrolimus)
    * Others (for example, azathioprine, mycophenolate mofetil, or rifamycin)

    Because of the side effects of the immunosuppression medications, patients are also prescribed:
    * H2 blockers
    * *Pneumocystis carinii* pneumonia (PCP) prophylaxis
    * Oral candidiasis prophylaxis
    * Antiviral therapy
    * Multivitamin supplementation
    * Calcium supplementation
    * Magnesium supplementation

    Depending on the individual's postoperative course, other medications may include:
    * Antiarrhythmics
    * Hypoglycemic agents
    * Antihypertensives
    * Anxiolytics
    * Narcotics
    * Anticoagulants

    And, of course, maintenance therapy for preexisting conditions is continued as needed.

21. **What are common side effects of post-transplant immunosuppression medications?**

    Calcineurin inhibitors:
    * Headache, tremors
    * Renal insufficiency

- Hypertension
- Hyperlipidemia
- Gastric dysmotility
- Neuropathy

Corticosteroids:
- Osteoporosis
- Diabetes mellitus
- Weight gain
- Hyperlipidemia
- Gastritis or peptic ulcers
- Oral/esophageal candidiasis

Others:
- Bone marrow suppression, anemia, leukopenia
- Shingles, acne, increased rates of skin cancers
- Reactivation of latent viral illnesses
- Increased risk for community acquired pneumonias

22. Other than taking medications, what precautions should a lung transplant recipient follow to stay healthy?

- Monitor pulmonary function daily with a home spirometer
- Perform daily temperature checks and maintain ideal body weight
- Exercise regularly
- Eat nutritious foods
- Maintain good personal hygiene
- Keep scheduled office visits and follow-up care with lung transplant team
- Avoid infections (for example, minimize contacts with people in poor health, use fastidious hand-washing, practice safe sex)
- Immediately report any changes in health to transplant team
- Have teeth cleaned twice a year
- Maintain timely vaccinations against influenza and pneumococcal pneumonia
- Follow routine primary care (for example, colonoscopy, mammogram, PSA screening)

23. How are lung transplant recipients monitored for complications?

Though protocols vary from center to center, the standard follow-up regimen includes routine screening of quality of life measures, pulmonary function studies, chest radiography, functional status measurements (for example, 6-minute walk test, exercise study), and blood work that screens drug levels and general chemistries. Attention is paid to both absolute values and individual patient trends.

24. What are the common infections seen in lung transplant recipients?

Bacterial:
- Purulent bronchitis, bronchiectasis, pneumonia
  - Gram-negative pathogens (for example, *Pseudomonas aeruginosa*) are most common

Viral:
- Pneumonitis, gastritis, colitis, viremia, retinitis
  - Cytomegalovirus
  - Herpes simplex virus
  - Varicella zoster virus
  - Epstein-Barr virus

Fungal:
- Colonization versus invasive pulmonary disease
  - *Aspergillus fumigatus* most aggressive
  - *Candida* species

25. Why are infectious complications a major problem in lung transplantation?

Infection is a leading cause of death in lung transplant patients. Unlike other solid organ transplants, the allograft is exposed to the external environment with each breath, making it more susceptible to infection. In addition, immuno-suppression medication levels are higher to protect against a higher rate of rejection in lung transplant recipients, rendering these patients at increased risk for infection.

26. How is acute rejection diagnosed?

Patients may be asymptomatic with acute rejection or may exhibit symptoms such as dyspnea, malaise, and low-grade fever. Common clinical features include perihilar infiltrates on chest x-ray, reduction of forced vital capacity (FVC) and forced expiratory volume in 1 second (FEV_1) on spirometry, or reduction in oxygen saturation (SaO_2) at rest or with exertion. Definitive diagnosis is made with tissue biopsy of the allograft.

27. What are the clinical manifestations of chronic pulmonary allograft rejection?

Chronic rejection is manifested as bronchiolitis obliterans syndrome (BOS), a progressive obstructive lung disease characterized by fibroproliferation within the small airways. A recipient is labeled as having BOS when there is an otherwise unexplained and persistent loss of greater than 20% of lung function (FEV_1) from the best post-transplant values. Patients often report productive cough and worsening dyspnea leading to functional decline. Controversy exists as to the mechanism of this entity. To date there remains no cure for BOS. The aim of therapy is to slow disease progression.

28. What is the life expectancy following lung transplantation?

According to the Organ Procurement Transplant Network, data as of August 1, 2002 reflect the following survival rates among all recipients of cadaveric donor lungs:
- 3-month survival = 88.2% (standard error = 0.8%)
- 1-year survival = 77.4% (standard error = 1.0%)
- 3-year survival = 59.3% (standard error = 1.2%)
- 5-year survival = 42.5% (standard error = 1.3%)

Key Points

- Patients with septic lung disease require bilateral lung transplantation.
- The 1-year survival rate after lung transplantation is approximately 77%.
- The acceptable ischemic time for the donor lung is 4 to 6 hours.

 Internet Resources

United Network for Organ Sharing:
http://www.unos.org

Second Wind Lung Transplant Association:
http://www.2ndwind.org

The International Society for Heart and Lung Transplantation:
http://www.ishlt.org

BIBLIOGRAPHY

Alexander BD, Tapson VF: Infectious complications of lung transplantation, *Transplant Infect Dis* 3: 128-137, 2001.

Arcasoy SM, Kotloff RM: Lung transplantation, *N Engl J Med* 340:1081-1091, 1999.

Couture KA: *The Lung Transplantation Handbook*, ed 2, Victoria, British Columbia, 2001, Trafford.

Estenne M, Maurer JR, Boehler A, et al: Bronchiolitis obliterans syndrome 2001: an update of the diagnostic criteria, *J Heart Lung Transplant* 21:197-310, 2002.

Kuos PC, Schoeder RA, Johnson LB, editors: *Clinical Management of the Transplant Patient*, New York, 2001, Arnold.

Lubetkin EI, Lipson DA, Palevsky HI, et al: GI complications after orthotopic lung transplantation, *Am J Gastroenterol* 91:2382-2390, 1996.

Penn I: Posttransplant malignancies, *Transplant Proc* 31:1260-1262, 1999.

Spira A, Gutierrez C, Chaparro C, Hutcheon MA, Chan CK: Osteoporosis and lung transplantation: a prospective study, *Chest* 117:476-481, 2000.

Management of the Postoperative Thoracic Surgery Patient

Janice Jones

1. **What are potential intraoperative complications during pulmonary resection?**

One complication is injury to a major blood vessel, resulting in massive hemorrhage. If this occurs during a video-assisted thoracoscopy (VATS) procedure, the surgery may need to progress to either a thoracotomy or a median sternotomy. The patient may also develop a contralateral pneumothorax. This is a higher risk in patients with bullous lung disease and emphysema. Spinal cord injury rarely occurs, but is usually the result of attempts to control persistent intercostal bleeding.

2. **What are some general principles of management during the postoperative period?**

Prevention and early detection of postoperative problems is essential. Patients should be assessed at least once a day. Removal of all tubes and catheters as soon as possible, early mobilization, close monitoring of fluid and electrolyte balance, and adequate pain control are imperative for good nursing care.

3. **What are the main findings that should be assessed on a postpneumonectomy chest x-ray?**

Tracheal position should be studied, making sure the trachea is midline. Over the next few days, it is imperative to evaluate the chest for fluid buildup. The side of the pneumonectomy should fill with serosanguineous fluid. This can take anywhere from 2 weeks to a few months. The fluid within the space is gradually absorbed. Complete absorption is uncommon.

4. **Describe postoperative management of the pleural space after lobectomy or bullectomy.**

Postoperatively, these procedures require drainage. Two chest tubes are placed: one to drain air and the other to drain fluid. The tubes are usually left in the patient for a few days until reexpansion of the lung occurs. Some patients may have a persistent asymptomatic space, particularly patients with emphysema or bullectomy. At the time of surgery, if it is felt a space will be present, a pleural drain can be placed.

5. What are methods of pain control for the postoperative thoracic surgery patient?

Many patients will have the anesthesiologist place a thoracic epidural catheter preoperatively for pain control. These catheters will remain in place for approximately 2 to 3 days. Patients may also undergo cryoablation of the nerves near the incision site. This will numb the area; however, cryoablation has an effect that persists long after the surgery. Postoperative pain can also be managed by patient-controlled analgesia (PCA). This allows the patient to control medication administration. Once a patient is taking oral fluids and is nearing discharge, oral analgesics are administered. These can be narcotics, nonsteroidal antiinflammatory drugs, or acetaminophen. Some patients may have pain months to years later. This chronic thoracotomy pain syndrome can be managed by a pain control center.

6. What are general indications for chest tube placement?

Chest tubes can be placed for many reasons. Some more common indications are postoperative treatment of pneumothorax, pleural effusion, and empyema.

7. What is the basic setup for chest tubes?

Chest tubes have a three-chamber system: a collection chamber for blood and fluid; an underwater seal that allows air to be evacuated during expiration but not reintroduced during inspiration; and a wall suction chamber that regulates the amount of vacuum. This setup is used for all chest tubes except postpneumonectomy patients: pneumonectomy chest tubes do not have a chamber that connects to suction.

8. When managing chest tubes, what factors should be considered?

Chest tubes are used to evacuate air, fluid, or purulent drainage from the pleural space. When placed postoperatively, generally two chest tubes are used, one for air and one for fluid. Not all chest tubes are connected to wall suction. Postoperatively, it is the preference of the surgeon if the tubes should be connected to wall suction or water seal. Wall suction maintains negative intrathoracic pressure to keep the lung expanded. After a resection, once the lung has completely reexpanded, the tubes can be placed to water seal and then discontinued.

9. What is the implication of "bubbling" in the water chamber of a chest tube?

When an air leak is present, there will be "bubbling" in the water chamber with respiration or coughing. If an air leak is present it may be necessary to continue the chest tube for days to weeks until the air leak is resolved. If these air leaks do not resolve spontaneously, as is common in patients with emphysema, the patient may need to have surgical intervention. If there is a continuous air leak, "bubbling" persisting in the chamber, it is important to check all connections of the chest tube and to determine placement of the chest tube within the chest. It should be determined if all holes of the chest tube itself are within the thoracic cavity and if all connections are secure.

10. **What factors contribute to the morbidity and mortality associated with thoracic surgery?**

There are many factors that contribute to the morbidity and mortality associated with thoracic surgery. The general physical status of the patient and comorbid factors can contribute to the patient's risk. Measurement of pulmonary function tests and arterial blood gas can indicate a patient's prognosis from a pulmonary standpoint. The nature of the pathologic process also contributes to the risk associated with surgery. The extent of the procedure and the addition of preoperative or postoperative adjunctive therapy can also affect outcomes.

11. **Describe the cause and treatment for hemorrhage after thoracic surgery.**

Postoperative hemorrhage is most commonly associated with inadequate hemostasis of bronchial vessels in the chest wall. If chest tube output is generally greater than 200 ml/hr, this is usually indicative of the need for reexploration. Another indication of hemorrhage is opacification of the ipsilateral thorax as seen on chest x-ray. If bleeding from a major pulmonary vessel is the problem, the first indication may be syncope and hypotension with failure to respond to fluids. This is an emergency situation requiring reexploration.

12. **What is a common cardiac complication seen after thoracic surgery?**

Cardiac dysrhythmias are typical complications of lobectomy and pneumonectomy. Atrial fibrillation and flutter is the most common cardiac complication and can occur postlobectomy with a 15% to 20% incidence and postpneumonectomy with a 20% to 30% incidence. The cause of this complication is unknown and usually occurs within 7 days. The prevalence is increased with age, cardiac disease, and complexity of the procedure. The most common treatment for atrial arrhythmia is the use of digoxin, calcium channel blockers, or beta-blockers. Dependent on the degree of lung pathology, beta-blockers and amiodarone may be contraindicated.

13. **What is the importance of early mobilization in the postoperative patient?**

Early mobilization is extremely important postoperatively in all patients; however, it may be even more vital in the postoperative thoracic surgery patient. A very typical complication of surgery is the development of atelectasis and pneumonia. In a patient with lung disease, the respiratory reserve is decreased when the injury of pulmonary infection is added. These patients, who may not breath deeply or move secondary to pain, retain secretions and lack proper aeration of their lungs. Providing adequate pain control that allows the patient to get out of bed as soon as possible and resume walking lowers the chance of developing pneumonia. Another reason for early mobilization is to decrease the incidence of pulmonary embolism. Remaining bed-bound postoperatively increases the risk of deep venous thrombosis (DVT) development. DVTs can become dislodged and cause thrombosis to the lung, a potentially devastating complication.

14. What is subcutaneous emphysema?

Subcutaneous emphysema is air trapped within the pleural space; it is not adequately drained by a chest tube, if present. The air is forced out through the surgical incision within the rib cage into the soft tissues. This will cause a "crackling" sound upon palpation. The only treatment is to improve existing means of drainage or to secure a new pathway to drain air.

15. How is a pneumothorax detected and treated postoperatively?

In the thoracic surgery patient a chest x-ray is usually checked daily, at least while the chest tube is present. The chest x-ray is the most common way to detect a pneumothorax. Some indications that a pneumothorax may be present are increasing respiratory difficulty and a sharp pain that is present on the affected side. Some pneumothoraces may be asymptomatic. Treatment varies depending on many factors. The size of the pneumothorax is important. A small pneumothorax may be treated with oxygen alone. Larger pneumothoraces usually require further intervention. If a chest tube is present from surgery, and is on water seal, you may need to return it to wall suction. If the chest tube is currently on wall suction, check the function of the chest tube. If there is no chest tube present, one may need to be placed.

16. What is the treatment for an empyema?

The development of an empyema is a known complication of thoracic surgery. On chest x-ray a loculated pleural effusion will be found. If this is associated with fever, bacteremia, and difficulty with pulmonary function, an empyema should be suspected. Initially a chest tube is placed for drainage. If the lung reexpands, the tube can be removed; however, many empyemas, particularly chronic ones, have a thick wall and need to be surgically treated. In this instance an empyema tube is left in place, cut at the level of the skin, and allowed to drain. Slowly over weeks to months the cavity will close behind the tube, gently pushing it out of the thoracic cavity. Because of the nature of the cavity and the usual widespread pleural adhesions, a pneumothorax usually does not develop.

17. What are other less common, but potential complications of thoracic surgery?

There are many other complications that can occur after thoracic surgery. A chylothorax can develop. A chylothorax is the result of injury to the thoracic duct.

It is manifested by a change in the character of chest tube drainage to a milky fluid. This injury can slowly heal spontaneously, but often requires surgical repair. An esophageal injury can also occur. This is usually the result of dissection close to the area of the esophagus. This injury may lead to a fistula, which in turn can cause mediastinitis or an empyema.

18. **What is a tension pneumothorax?**

A tension pneumothorax is a life-threatening condition caused by increasingly positive pleural pressure with respect to the atmospheric pressure. When this occurs the mediastinum can shift to the opposite side, impairing contralateral function and systemic venous return. This can arise from a simple pneumothorax, particularly if positive pressure ventilation is being used. Treatment is release of the air from the pleural space, allowing the mediastinum to return to center. This is an emergent situation.

19. **Postoperatively, how can pulmonary function be maximized?**

Pulmonary function can be maximized in many ways. Providing adequate pain control is very important. Thoracic surgery incisions, which go through the rib spaces, are painful with each breath. Providing adequate pain control will allow the patient to take deep breaths. Early mobilization is also very important. Early movement allows patients to breath deeper, cough easier, and decrease the risk of development of DVTs. The use of an incentive spirometer is also needed. This will aid in the expansion of the alveoli, helping in the removal of secretions. Nebulizer treatments can also be useful, particularly in patients with asthma or chronic obstructive pulmonary disease (COPD).

 Key Points

- Early mobilization is key to the prevention of complications after thoracic surgery.
- Chylothorax is the result of injury to the thoracic duct.
- Atrial fibrillation can occur in nearly 30% of patients undergoing thoracic surgery.

 Internet Resources

The New England Journal of Medicine: Randomized Trial Comparing Lung-Volume-Reduction Surgery with Medical Therapy in Severe Emphysema:
http://www.nejm.org/cgi/content/abstract/NEJMoa030287v1

AllRefer.com: Health: Surgeries and Procedures:
http://www.AllRefer.com.Health:LungSurgery

BIBLIOGRAPHY

Baumgartner FJ: *Cardiothoracic Surgery, 1997,* RG Landes and Chapman & Hall, New York.

Criner GJ, D'Alonzo G: *Pulmonary Pathophysiology,* Madison, Connecticut 1999, Fence Creek.

Ewald GA, McKenzie CR, editors: *Manual of Medical Therapeutics,* ed 28, 1995, Boston, Little, Brown and Company.

Index

A

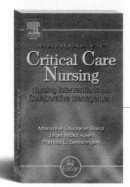